D1255566

Southern Biography Series
William J. Cooper, Jr., Editor

WAR
AND
HEALING

WAR
AND
HEALING

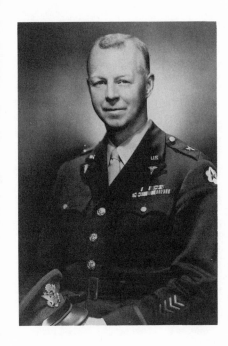

STANHOPE BAYNE-JONES
AND THE MATURING
OF AMERICAN MEDICINE

ALBERT E. COWDREY

LOUISIANA STATE UNIVERSITY PRESS
Baton Rouge and London

01 00 99 98 97 96 95 94 93 92   5 4 3 2 1

Designer: G. Phoebe
Typeface: Caledonia
Typesetter: G&S Typesetters, Inc.
Printer and binder: Thomson-Shore, Inc.

Library of Congress Cataloging-in-Publication Data
Cowdrey, Albert E.
    War and healing : Stanhope Bayne-Jones and the maturing of
American medicine / Albert E. Cowdrey
        p.   cm.—(Southern biography series)
    Includes bibliographical references and index.
    ISBN 0-8071-1717-X (cloth : alk. paper)
    1. Bayne-Jones, Stanhope, 1888–1970.   2. Physicians—United
States—Biography.   I. Title.   II. Series.
    [DNLM: 1. Bayne-Jones, Stanhope, 1888–1970.   2. History of
Medicine—United States.   3. Physicians—biography.   WZ 100 B3617C]
R154.B336C68   1991
610'.92—dc20
[B]
DNLM/DLC
for Library of Congress   91-32513
                                                                     CIP

Portrait on title page of Stanhope Bayne-Jones as a general in the United States Army
Medical Corps, 1945, courtesy of Bachrach Studios and the National Library of Medicine

To George Denegre II, who asked only for the truth

Contents

Illustrations

New Orleans–born Stanhope Bayne-Jones was one of the most influential American doctors of the twentieth century. A man of science who pursued power, a doctor who plunged into war with relish, and a soldier who saved countless lives, he embodied well the unaccountable variety of life, the subject of the medical art.

To his formidable array of friends and acquaintances he was B-J, a coinage that seemed to imply both informality and distance, as if he were a chairman of the board, pleased to be called by his initials. In fact, people responded to him with deference as well as warmth. He was willful as well as kind, rough beneath his geniality, often alone and guarded despite his cheerful sociability. Through a remarkable collection of papers and memorabilia he left behind, the reader gains insight not only into his complex character, but into an extraordinary variety of events in medicine, government, and war—medical support at the battle of Passchendaele, the inner workings of Yale's School of Medicine, the American biological warfare program, and the inner history of the Surgeon General's Commission on Smoking and Health, to name a few.

The fusing of personal and historical events in part reflects the fact that B-J's life paralleled the growth of American medicine from a provincial and amateurish state to a major national endeavor. Spurred by the wars of the twentieth century, government became the greatest patron of science and medicine. Academic physicians rose on the great research wave, first accepting foundation grants and then, in some cases, leading the foundations that gave them. Many moved easily into quasi-governmental bodies and the agencies of government. They influenced the military that employed many of them and were in turn influenced by wartime imperatives.

Bayne-Jones followed that path, toward not only influence and power but an increasingly broad conception of an ideal medicine that would be free of political control, devoted to the preservation of health, organized collectively, and divorced from entrepreneurial passions. But he was also part of the process by which medicine became rich at the cost of submitting to the many uses that those in power might find for it. He was both a unique and a representative figure, and I hope that this account may help to rescue from obscurity a man and physician who deserves to be more widely known.

Writing a book has its lonely moments. But the process also involves many human contacts and causes the writer to incur a variety of debts to the people who assist him along the way. This book began with George Denegre II, whose wish for an objective history of his uncle's life led him to John Duffy, dean of this nation's medical historians, and to Robert J. T. Joy, M.D., a leading authority on the history of military medicine. They directed him to me, and because I had already encountered Bayne-Jones frequently in my earlier researches into American military medicine, I was glad to accept the challenge.

My way in resolving the complex research problems that ensued was greatly assisted by the generosity of the Eugenie and Joseph Jones Family Foundation of New Orleans. The daunting scope of the Bayne-Jones collection at the National Library of Medicine had begun to make me feel that I might never work my way through it, when my appointment as visiting scholar for six months in 1985 and 1986 suddenly smoothed the whole process by enabling me to work with the papers all day, every day. For this opportunity I am indebted not only to John Parascandola, chief of the Medical History Division of the library, but also to Maj. Gen. William A. Stofft, then chief of military history, who allowed me to accept the offer.

Two of Bayne-Jones's friends and younger colleagues were especially helpful in providing valuable insights into the man and his time: Thomas B. Turner, M.D., dean emeritus of the Johns Hopkins University School of Medicine, who granted a lengthy interview, and Tom F. Whayne, Sr., M.D., to whose rigorous and insightful critique of the final manuscript I owe much. Edward F. Adolph, M.D., of the University of Rochester Medical Center, shared papers of Bayne-Jones's along with undimmed recollections of events more than sixty years in the past. Members of Bayne-Jones's family were no less helpful, especially George Denegre II, Thomas B. and Louise Denegre, and Nenette Denegre Keenan. Joy and Duffy provided penetrating criticisms of the manuscript, as did my colleague at the army's Center of Military History, Mary C. Gillett.

My debts to resident historians, archivists, and librarians in many repositories are particularly great. At the National Library of Medicine I was privileged to associate with James Cassedy and James Harvey Young, two of our premier medical historians, during my stay. Philip Teigen, Dorothy Hanks, Margaret Kaiser, and Karen Pitts were all unfailingly helpful. Harold Kanarek of the Alan Mason Chesney Medical Archives at Johns Hopkins provided me knowledgeable assistance.

I owe my thanks for similar assistance to Judith Ann Schiff and the staff of the Department of Manuscripts and Archives at Yale's Sterling Memorial Library, and to Ferenc Gyorgyey of the Historical Library, Yale Medical Library. Richard Boylan and Will Mahoney of the National Archives displayed their customary omniscience regarding the records under their care. Adele Lerner of the Samuel J. Wood Library, Cornell University Medical College, courteously made its rich and well-organized holdings available to me during an agreeable visit to New York. The staffs of the Tulane University and Louisiana State University archives and the Louisiana Room of the New Orleans Public Library were no less helpful; I regret that my notes of specific names have disappeared.

Others to whom thanks are due include Harris D. Riley, Jr., M.D., who commented on an early draft; Mark L. Baker, who served briefly as contract researcher; and James Polk Morris, who, though prevented by circumstances from writing Bayne-Jones's biography, has retained a scholarly interest in the man and his work. But I would be less than generous to all those who have contributed to this work if I did not conclude by taking upon myself full responsibility for any errors and omissions that may still mar it.

Abbreviations

ABJS   Amelia Bayne Jones
Succession, Louisiana
Room, New Orleans Public
Library, New Orleans

AFEB   Armed Forces
Epidemiological Board

AMC   Allan M. Chesney Medical
Archives, Johns Hopkins
University, Baltimore

CCJP   Charles C. Jones Papers,
Louisiana State University
Archives, Baton Rouge

CMH   U.S. Army Center of
Military History,
Washington, D.C.

GDC   George Denegre II
Collection, New Orleans

JJP   Joseph Jones Papers,
Louisiana State University
Archives, Baton Rouge

MANY   Medical Archives, New
York Hospital–Cornell
University Medical Center,
New York

ABBREVIATIONS

NARA   National Archives and
           Records Administration,
           Washington, D.C.

NLM   National Library of
           Medicine, Bethesda,
           Maryland

RG   Record Group

SBJC   Stanhope Bayne-Jones
           Collection, National Library
           of Medicine

SBJT   Stanhope Bayne-Jones
           Collection, Tulane
           University Archives, New
           Orleans

SML   Sterling Memorial Library,
           Yale University, New
           Haven, Connecticut

WAR
AND
HEALING

ONE

Heritage

The hyphen told the story. Stanhope Bayne-Jones, physician, scientist, educator, soldier, came not of one family but two. Both belonged to the nineteenth-century American equivalent of a squirearchy, a comfortable middle class rooted in land, the officer corps, and the learned professions—the clergy, medicine, and law. Specifically, they belonged to the southern branch of that class, with its black slaves, its country ways, and, when the Civil War came, its experience of Confederate service, defeat, and damaged fortunes.[1]

In the years after Appomattox, Dr. Joseph Jones settled in New Orleans with his second wife and his five children, and embarked anew upon the practice of medicine. He was a complex man, a child of the Renaissance born too late or a scientist born too early. Fascinated by research, he lived at a time when a science of medicine was only beginning to take form. He suffered too from an encyclopedic inclusiveness, hankering to comprehend all things and, perhaps as a consequence, never achieving any single great discovery.[2]

Yet he performed some notable services. As a Confederate surgeon and medical inspector he wrote a report on Andersonville prison that became a primary source of information on that abominable place. In the aftermath of the war he served his adopted city as president of the Louisiana state board of health, making himself an important local figure in the new science of keeping people well. He prospered modestly, becoming a fixture on the medical faculty of the University of Louisiana—soon to be Tulane—and readily combined teaching with the practice of medicine. Research continued to claim his off-hours, and

1. Robert Manson Myers, ed., *The Children of Pride* (abr. ed., New Haven, 1984), 662–63. Discussion of the Jones family is condensed here, in view of the exhaustive treatment available in Myers' work.

2. James O. Breeden, *Joseph Jones, M.D.: Scientist of the Old South* (Lexington, Ky., [1975]); Paul Starr, *The Social Transformation of American Medicine* (New York, 1982), 81ff.; John Duffy, *The Healers: A History of American Medicine* (Urbana, 1976), 166–88.

he followed with intense interest the birth of scientific medicine then taking place in European laboratories.[3]

In the 1880s his oldest son, Samuel Stanhope Davis Jones, won the post of valedictorian of the 1883 graduating class in medicine at the University of Louisiana. A handsome youth with straw-blond hair, Stanhope (as he was always called) found research as entrancing as his father did. He found it equally hard to finance, however, and soon went into practice, charging his patients about two dollars a visit.[4]

Sometime in the winter of 1885 to 1886, he met Amelia Elizabeth Bayne, known as Minna. She was eighteen, a spirited and engaging young woman who had excellent financial prospects. Almost penniless, but with a respectable profession and standing in the community, the young doctor soon began to take more than a passing interest in Minna, and she in him.

The Baynes, too, had moved from the country to the city. They, too, belonged to the professional class. Their field was law.

Thomas Levingston Bayne was a native of Georgia who, fortified by a Yale education, moved in 1843 to New Orleans, where he read law and entered the firm of Slidell & Clarke. Soon he was made a partner. In December, 1853, he married Maria, a daughter of former governor John Gayle of Alabama. The Civil War sent him first to the battle of Shiloh, where he was severely wounded, and later to Richmond. Maria Gayle's sister Amelia had married General Josiah Gorgas, the Confederate chief of ordnance. (Their son, William Crawford Gorgas, later became surgeon general of the United States Army.) Commissioned, Bayne rose rapidly from a job under Gorgas to the rank of lieutenant colonel and chief of the bureau of foreign supplies, a post of importance in a government obliged to fight its war of independence so largely with materiel run through the blockade. When the war ended, he returned to New Orleans. He estimated his worth at about five thousand dollars;

---

3. Breeden has in preparation a second volume on Joseph Jones's life after the Civil War. See also Stanhope Bayne-Jones, *Joseph Jones* (N.p., [1957]).
4. New Orleans *Daily States*, March 29, 1883; see also Stanhope Jones's thesis, "The Microscope," in A-18, Box 3, SBJC.

by the time of his death, in 1891, he would have increased it just about one hundred times over.[5]

The sixties were abysmal, the seventies hard in New Orleans. But the firm Bayne had joined, which was now called Clarke, Bayne & Renshaw, survived and in 1880 made twenty-six-year-old George Denegre a partner. Concealing a sharp mind under an unimpressive exterior, Denegre was a product of bilingual creole New Orleans. His family had been exiled from the city during the regime of General Benjamin Butler; he had been educated in Brussels, Belgium, and later at Fordham and the University of Louisiana. In 1882 Denegre married Minna Bayne's sister Edith. A convivial clubman, a cautious and competent lawyer, he trod warily in the presence of his vivid and emphatic wife while building their fortune and gradually assuming leadership of the clan.[6]

By 1880 the hard years of war and depression were fading. For the Baynes, Denegres, and Joneses, New Orleans must have been a pleasant place as it revived after twenty years of upheaval. The fashionable district was now far Uptown, along St. Charles Avenue and its side streets, where comfortable houses multiplied amid semitropical greenery and deep sward. Not only comfort but health improved. In 1878 the city had suffered 4,000 yellow fever deaths from a population of less than 200,000. But two years later it had a determined board of health and, in Dr. Jones, a courageous leader who quarantined ships with little regard to the complaints of merchants. A new association of progressive businessmen set to work, aiding the effort to prevent disease.

As in the past, civic corruption was the norm; illness and poverty abounded. But the Baynes and the Joneses—like much of their community—faced the future with new confidence as Stanhope Jones and Minna Bayne entered the throes of courtship.[7]

5. See Thomas L. Bayne's Letter to His Children, October 6, 1870, A-9, and Brief Sketch of the Lives of Hugh Gayle Bayne's Bayne Progenitors, A-8, both in Box 1, SBJC. Hugh Gayle Bayne was one of Thomas L. Bayne's grandsons.

6. See items in A-9, Box 1, SBJC.

7. Hugh A. Bayne, Memoirs, Vol. I, 137, 180–81, in SML. For background on New Orleans, see Joy Jackson, *New Orleans in the Gilded Age: Politics and Urban Progress, 1880–1896* (Baton Rouge, 1969), 88, 90–91, 93, 96, 145, 149–50, 171–72, 231.

How they met is uncertain, but they belonged to the same class in a small, clubby city. On February 23, 1886, Stanhope invited Minna in the third person to confer "the honor of dancing with him the 'Carnival German.'" Minna declined. From this point matters developed with deliberate speed.[8]

By May, he was sending her simpering verse clipped from magazines. (Verse, sentimental or comic, was a hobby with him; he both collected and wrote it.) The early phases of the relationship were stilted, enveloped in formalized Victorian sentiment. ("Am I lonely? Do I miss you? Why My Dear Miss Minna: The realization eclipses conception.")[9] Whether the romance was serious at this point was probably unclear to the parties most concerned, and remains so.

Then Minna left the city for a summer of travel. Separation brought a note of anguish into his unanswered notes. By the end of July he was writing, "It seems to me I live just to love you," and by mid-August he was leaving New Orleans to join her. They spent time together in Narragansett and Boston, where he apparently proposed and she, in timeless fashion, put him on probation. There was little doubt who was in charge, the twenty-five-year-old doctor or the eighteen-year-old girl. Her return home in October set off a flurry of hand-delivered notes to the Bayne home, most intended to supplement or confirm what Stanhope was saying in person. He reasoned and pleaded; he quoted the sonnet, "Let me not to the marriage of true minds / Admit impediments"; he spoke of his thriving practice. He brought "pretty microscopical specimens" to the house on St. Joseph Street, and they viewed them together.[10]

Minna said yes on January 28, 1887, succumbing gracefully after an exciting siege. Thomas L. Bayne promptly gave his consent, almost depriving Stanhope of the ability to gush. With true Victorian deliberation, the family fixed the wedding date for the following autumn. They were "united in marriage by Father Hubert" on November 15, 1887, in the house on St. Joseph Street, "exquisitely decorated" for the occa-

8. Stanhope Jones to Minna Bayne, February 22, 1886, in A-22, Box 4, SBJC. The story of the courtship is in this source.

9. Stanhope Jones to Minna Bayne, [June 24?] 1886, *ibid*.

10. Stanhope Jones to Minna Bayne, August 6 [postmark], 1886, September 6, 1886, *ibid*.; "microscopical specimens" mentioned in Stanhope to Minna, n.d., *ibid*.

sion. They went to live on Howard Avenue near recently christened Lee Circle, a property that Thomas L. Bayne had given to Minna. Their first child was born on November 6, 1888, a son whom they named Stanhope.[11]

"Well," wrote Minna's sister Edith to her younger brother Hugh, then away at school, "the great event is over & Minna has a fat little son. It all passed off in 2 ½ hours with the dignity, quietude & elegance which characterizes the Bayne family, especially Mrs. Jones. The little one we thought dead for a few minutes & [he] had to be violently slapped, plunged into cold water, [and] have ice applied. With his first cry he was given a drink of whiskey & thank God revived. . . . Poor little fellow he is so sore he screams all the time, but it is music to know for sure he is alive & strong with great lung power. Monsieur was born at 2.20 & at three Min would have liked to get up to dinner." The infant's few hairs were fiery red, and he weighed in at seven and a half pounds.[12] On March 12, 1890, a daughter followed and was named Marian Gayle Jones.

Minna gloried in her children. "Little Stanhope no longer talks— he converses," she confided to a friend in June, 1890. He knew "Mother Hubbard" and "Rain, rain, go away." Proudly she reported the first signs of the fearlessness that was to be so marked a part of his character. He climbed the attic stairs, announcing that he wanted to see the darkness that lingered there all day. "Everything is a living and friendly presence to him—when he comes down from the attic he says, 'Good-bye dark, I goin' down-stairs now.'" He came to know his grandfather Jones's house in addition to his own. In 1891 Joseph Jones had a Christmas tree for a company of children that included Stanhope and Marian. He was "perfectly wild with delight, and wanted to take the tree home with him."[13]

11. Undated notes [by one of the Jones aunts?] on "Stanhope Jones, M.D." letterhead, in A-24, Box 6, SBJC.
12. Edith Bayne Denegre to Hugh Aiken Bayne, November 7, 1888, and "few hairs" mentioned in Mary Vaught to Hugh Bayne, November 9, 1888, both in A-23, Box 6, SBJC.
13. Minna Bayne Jones to Carrie [not identified], June 1, 1890, July 20, 1890, in GDC; Frances Devereux Jones to Charles C. Jones, December 29, 1891, in Box 2, Folder 1, CCJP.

At home, the sick and injured were familiar sights to the boy. Less than two years old, but babbling freely in a way his mother thought *"truly wonderful,"* he watched his father work over a broken limb and reported to his nursemaid, "Mammy, old woman break her leg, Papa fix it *now!"* In the dispensary, he performed his first medical task, winding bandages. The doctor had a homemade device for this, "a kind of twisted, angular wire over a cigar box," and Stanhope, Jr., learned to turn a crank to roll the bandages on the wire.[14]

It was all part of the "very happy sort of a beginning" he enjoyed in the house on Howard Avenue. There were also trips outside the city, when Edith (whom he called Tante E) took him to her house, Malua, on the Mississippi gulf coast. Here Stanhope, Jr., sailed and fished and played in the fine white sand, absorbing scenes that lingered at the back of his mind throughout life—the galleried houses, the piling cumuli, the summer days of exquisite heat.[15]

Perhaps Stanhope Jones was too conscious of the fact that he lived in his wife's house. Though he labored hard and long at his profession, his work was not enough to bring him independent wealth. On the other hand, a successful investment might.

His younger brother Charles (Charlie, to the family) was a mining engineer, as well educated and lacking in wealth as he. Working amid the coalfields of southwestern Virginia, Charlie piqued Stanhope's interest with an invitation to join him in the risks and possible rewards of founding their own company. Stanhope and Minna spent the summer of 1892 among the cool hills near Lynchburg. By now she was pregnant again, and her husband's urge to find financial reinforcement correspondingly increased. The brothers rode often together; the children and Minna were happy, and all returned to New Orleans in blooming condition. Minna noted that Stanhope, Sr., was "intensely interested"

14. Minna Bayne Jones to Carrie, June 1, 1890, GDC; Stanhope Bayne-Jones, interviews with Harlan B. Phillips, Bethesda, Md., 1967, p. 3, NLM (hereinafter cited as Phillips interview).

15. Phillips interview, 4; Sarah Jones to Stanhope Jones, March 2, 1893, in A-24, Box 6, SBJC. *Malua* is apparently a Polynesian word meaning gently, slowly, quietly, or by-and-by. The house was destroyed by Hurricane Camille in 1969.

in the mining venture, and could talk of nothing but their summer journey.[16]

He began investing heavily, living with the anxiety of a man who bets beyond his means. Meanwhile, as winter approached, Minna had much to do; her coming confinement occupied her thoughts. Stanhope and Marian were moved out of the nursery; Minna's sister Edith brought her a "magnificent baby-basket from N.Y.," and one of her sisters-in-law gave her a silver box for diaper pins. Making clothing for the child to come, she dreamed of having another girl, and decided to name it Millicent.

Sensing that something was afoot, Stanhope, Jr., followed his mother everywhere—"he sticks to me like a postage-stamp," Minna complained. If she rose to get a spool of thread, he followed her; if she drove him away, he sat outside the door of the room and wept. But when he was in bed his parents enjoyed quiet times together. Minna liked to read aloud to her husband (though she told a friend that a story entitled "The Suicide Club" gave them both nightmares).[17]

She gave birth to a boy, subsequently named Thomas Bayne Jones, on January 18, 1893, with her husband in attendance. No record survives to indicate whether the birth was easy or difficult, but puerperal fever soon appeared. Despite Stanhope's frantic efforts, the infection spread and developed into septicemia. In mid-February Stanhope wrote to his sister Susie a "wild burst of grief and anxiety over Minna's critical danger." Otherwise he controlled his emotions as well as he could, his face white and full of "infinite suffering."[18]

By the last week of February Minna was on opiates to dull the pain; her pulse was weak, and though she was still conscious, her wits wandered. In moments of clarity she attempted to make reasonable arrangements for her children. Her husband's household was to stay together; his sisters, Susan and Mary—Aunt Susie and Aunt Mamie to the children—would move in to care for them all. When she was dying,

16. Minna Jones to Charles C. Jones, October 24, 1892, in Box 2, Folder 1, CCJP.

17. Minna Bayne Jones to Carrie, December 2, 1892, in GDC; Minna Bayne Jones to Charles C. Jones, October 24, 1892, in Box 2, Folder 2, CCJP.

18. Susan Jones to Charles C. Jones, February 12, 1893, in Box 2, Folder 4, CCJP; postcard, Frances Jones to Charles C. Jones, in Box 2, Folder 7, CCJP. Puerperal fever is usually a result of contamination of the uterine lining; common sources of contamination at this time were unclean hands and unclean instruments.

Minna called for her brother Hugh to stand by the foot of the bed and whistle tunes that she knew. She died sometime on March 2, 1893.

Within a week of Minna's death George Denegre opened the succession, and Stanhope's extraordinary legal situation became clear. Minna, young and vigorous, had left no will, and during her illness neither her husband nor her family of lawyers had persuaded her to make one. In consequence, under Louisiana law all her property went to her children—more than $60,000 in real estate and notes. The Civil District Court intervened, appointing Stanhope tutor of his children and administrator of Minna's property in their behalf. He now inhabited a house owned by his children; he ate from his children's table; and the eldest, Stanhope, Jr., was four.[19]

A trap was closing about the young father. In the same month that Minna died, a financial panic plunged the nation into depression. No account books exist to reveal the condition of Stanhope's practice, but doctors suffered during hard times, unable to refuse care to patients who paid first their bills for food and lodging and put the doctor's aside. Stanhope tried to borrow on his stock in Charlie's mining enterprise, but no one in New Orleans knew anything of it, and no one would lend. By May he was writing to his brother that the success of the venture was his last hope. "This is the last straw to the drowning man—the last resort as it were—" But Charlie was mining coal for eighty-seven cents a ton and selling it for seventy-five. "Very discouraging," Stanhope admitted.[20]

To anyone who did not know his problems, things seemed to go well enough, or as well as possible with Minna gone. At home, his "ferocious little ones" were healthy. When the school in Philadelphia where Susie and Mamie were teaching closed for the summer, they gratefully returned south. Though Mamie was later to marry while Susie became a confirmed spinster, it was Susie who most successfully mothered the children. Stanhope, Jr., felt closest to her of all the array of aunts and uncles who would soon rule his life—"a very lovely person who, I think, cared for me a great deal."[21]

19. The legal situation may be followed in Doc. No. 38,367, Civil District Court, Division C, ABJS.

20. Stanhope Jones to Charles C. Jones, May 31, 1893, in Box 2, Folder 4, CCJP.

21. C. S. Jones [Susan] to Charles C. Jones, January 26, 1891, in Box 2, Folder 1, CCJP; Phillips interview, 7.

The year 1893 continued in the dismal way it had begun. Joseph Jones suffered his second stroke, and Susie and Mamie divided their time between the two stricken households. Then a bank in Abingdon, Virginia, that had been financing Charlie's schemes went under, and in August the coal company failed. With the bank in receivership, creditors turned on the brothers. "Every pressure will now be brought to bear on us," the young doctor noted, adding that the "added responsibility . . . threatens my annihilation."[22]

The situation was worse than even Charlie knew. Surviving records indicate that Stanhope had been going into debt since 1890, maintaining his family's comfortable lifestyle by borrowing from Peter to pay Paul. By 1893 he already owed at least $25,000. Even the money he invested in the mine had been borrowed. Among Minna's assets were promissory notes, some of which Stanhope had used during her lifetime as security for loans. Now he turned to them again. On one, with a face value of $14,250, he borrowed $27,000 from two different lenders. And there were other notes belonging to his children on which he also borrowed.[23]

The court had appointed T. L. Bayne, Jr., Minna's eldest living brother, as undertutor of the children. By autumn at the latest, T. L. had become aware of what was happening to the estate. In November he petitioned the court to remove Stanhope from the position of tutor and to appoint himself instead. Confronted with evidence of his wrongdoing, and possibly threatened with prosecution, Stanhope confessed. Duly the court deprived him of his tutorship, and with it the house, the furniture, everything but his clothing and the tools of his trade. Unable to support his children, he surrendered them as well.

On November 27, a conference of the two families met. By their agreement, Stanhope, Jr., went to live with his grandfather Jones; the two younger children went to the Denegres, who were childless. In January, 1894, the court allowed T. L. to sell the house on

22. Stanhope Jones to Charles C. Jones, September 27, 1893, in CCJP. See also George Denegre to Dr. Chaillé, July 22, 1900, and Mary Jones to T. L. Bayne, October 3, 1894, both in A-24, Box 6, SBJC.

23. The situation emerges clearly in Stanhope's confession, in document labeled "Testimony Filed Nov. 20/93," in ABJS. Though the facts are clear enough, the question of whether fraud was committed is not; under Louisiana law a note must be delivered to the lender in order to be legally pledged.

Howard Avenue to settle debts and provide a larger legacy for the children.[24]

The rest of Stanhope, Sr.'s life is soon told. To be close to his children, he chose a boardinghouse on St. Charles Avenue, living in a "small little bedroom in the back ell of the house on the second floor." Then, hoping to recover his fortunes, he left town with his brother Charlie to look over the wreck of the property in Virginia. He died before 1894 was out, of dysentery, the family said. He was thirty-three.[25]

All of this left most bitter feelings. In the Bayne view, Stanhope, Sr., had misused his wife's property after failing, as attending physician, to save her life. Anger ran high on the other side as well. Even Joneses who acquiesced in Stanhope's downfall resented the Baynes' role in it. Among two families divided by an undying grievance, Stanhope Jones, Jr., five years old, would now live out the remainder of his childhood.

He entered his grandfather's house at the corner of Washington Avenue and Camp Street, the site of Christmas and Easter celebrations in the past, this time to live. If the mysterious processes of heredity had already marked him as a new and corrected edition of his grandfather—and in later years he was to discover uncanny similarities not merely in their interests but in their methods of research—then he was living in a house saturated with the man he would become.

A handsome neoclassic residence of stuccoed brick, the house had two stories, galleries for coolness, and embellishments of fine iron lace. Across the street stood a firehouse, with a fire engine and great horses that came plunging out at the shrilling of an electric bell. When Stanhope arrived, the Joneses were numerous. Joseph Jones lived with his second wife, Susan Polk Jones, daughter of Leonidas Polk, the warlike Episcopal bishop who had become a general in the Confederate army; with Susie and Mamie, sheltering after the debacle on Howard Avenue; and with Frances, Laura, and Hamilton Jones, the children of his sec-

24. Denegre to Chaillé, July 22, 1900, in A-24, Box 6, SBJC.

25. Phillips interview, 13. On the hostility between the families, see Mary Jones to T. L. Bayne, October 3, 1894, in A-24, Box 6, SBJC.

ond marriage. He had servants, of course—black maids, a cook, and a coachman.

Joseph Jones was now sixty-one, the unquestioned ruler of the house, but in manner dignified and soft-spoken. White-bearded, he dressed often in gray as became the Surgeon General of the United Confederate Veterans. Though partly paralyzed and older than his years, sensing perhaps that he had little time left, he kept at his profession of medicine. He had recovered sufficiently to ride in his buggy to Tulane, where he remained professor of chemistry and clinical medicine, and even to visit some patients. He ran a dispensary in his home, affording his grandson the pleasure of seeing some ghastly accident cases. As ever, the preoccupation of Joseph Jones's life was research, and he kept two laboratories.

But no single science could confine his interests. "The house," said Stanhope, still vividly aware of the place almost seventy years later, "was full of most strange things." There were Egyptian mummies, snakes preserved in all sorts of containers, and Indian remains— tomahawks, pipes, arrowheads, and bows—as well as swords, armor, Aztec relics, carved serpent heads, Hindu masks, and a basalt image of Vishnu. The library contained books in French and English, with much emphasis on travels and explorations in North America. But most of the books were by Joseph Jones. He had published his *Medical and Surgical Memoirs* at his own expense in four huge volumes, and all the second floor and part of the first were lined with bookshelves containing the unsold copies, "maybe thousands of them."[26]

For a boy, the exotic house was both fearful and fascinating. Sometimes he found it "ghost-like," full of shadows, and the grownups played on his fears to keep him quiet. One story they told him was curiously nightmarish and memorable: if he was bad, the moon would come down from the sky, catch him under the ribs with a pair of ice tongs, and carry him away. But there was too much in the house to tempt him. He tested the armor, donning a breastplate and persuading a friend to

26. Phillips interview, 2, 9. See also Joseph Jones, *Medical and Surgical Memoirs* . . . (New Orleans, 1876–90); *An Abstract of the Catalogue of the Archeological Collection of Joseph Jones, M.D., L.L.D., Preserved at His Residence, 1138 Washington Avenue, New Orleans, Louisiana* (New Orleans, 1911); and *Some Rare Books from the Library of Joseph Jones, M.D., L.L.D.* (New Orleans, n.d.). Copies of the catalogues in Box 17, Folder 136, JJP.

whack him with a two-handed sword. He tried an experiment in biology—poured coal oil on a goldfish pond in the yard and set it afire to see whether the fish could survive under a twelve-foot circle of flame. When the adults retaliated by locking him into a room, he found a supply of shotgun shells, patiently unloaded them, ran a trail of powder to a sunny spot under a window, and set it on fire with a magnifying glass. The powder flamed and hissed magnificently. "Shh—you know how it goes."[27]

Harassed by the noisy, hyperactive orphan, most of the adults spanked him. In the context of the time, he was not an abused child. But too many adults applied too many punishments, and the more he was beaten the worse he became. "I did a great many things that I don't look back on now with any pride," he was to say, "but they did punish me a good deal."[28]

Then in 1896 Joseph Jones died of a final stroke, the third parental figure the boy had lost in four years. The Joneses came on hard times; the old man's collections were broken up and sold, and Stanhope went to live with the Baynes.

He stayed with his guardian, T. L., and T. L.'s wife in a big French Quarter house with a courtyard. No longer the focus and burden of a houseful of adults, the boy was now "an extra" among the Baynes' three children. Then T. L. joined the Uptown migration, building a house next door to the residence of George Denegre and Edith. Here Stanhope, like his brother and sister, came under the influence of Minna's ailing sister and her astute creole husband.

Tante E was a small woman, petite when young, a wren in organdy; as she aged, she became stout, but she was at all times a dominating figure. Known in youth as "she who must be obeyed," she retained until death a passionate and demanding personality. "A very impulsive woman," Susie Jones judged her, "with an intense craving for the expression of affection,—which must often cause a certain agony to herself, as well as to other people."[29]

27. Phillips interview, 2–7.
28. *Ibid.*, 4–5.
29. *Ibid.*, 16; Susan Jones to Charles C. Jones, October 6, 1892, in GDC.

Her personal tragedy was an illness of unspecified nature, which, she later told Stanhope, was "the cause of my sterility." But Minna's death and the ruin of Stanhope, Sr., suddenly presented to Edith (and to George, no happier with childlessness than she) a miraculous opportunity. The Denegres had seen their plight, wrote Edith to Stanhope many years later, as a "mutual sorrow & misfortune, until you three children came to take the place of the dream children we longed for."[30]

No doubt the baby, Bayne, was the prize catch. He was male, and too young to remember anything of the mother whose death he had unwittingly caused, or of the father who had been cast out. Within a few years George changed the two children's surname to Denegre, though he did not formally adopt them. In Stanhope the Denegres seemed less interested. Nevertheless, Tante E became a great determining influence upon his life, deciding for the other adults and thus for him "where I'd go and what I did and when." Force of personality was not the only source of Edith's power. George Denegre was by far the ablest businessman of his generation in either family, and Edith ruled George, dramatizing her sufferings without stint.[31]

Under the Denegres' protection the children enjoyed many of the advantages of the wealthy. Then T. L., who had taken a leading role in punishing Stanhope, Sr., began to have financial problems of his own. He went bankrupt and had to leave New Orleans to repair his fortunes elsewhere. For a time Stanhope went to live with his favorite aunt, Susie Jones. But the Joneses were also in difficult circumstances, and Susie decided to return to her old job in Philadelphia, hoping to take Stanhope with her. The Baynes resisted—possession of the children had become a point of honor between the feuding clansmen.

Instead, when Susie left, Stanhope returned abruptly to his mother's family. He had no warning. One day, unaware that any changes were in the wind, he visited the Denegres to play with his brother and sister. After a time a little cart drove up, a black man guiding the horse. On the cart was a trunk and a small white iron bed—his trunk and his bed.[32] The Denegres had gathered in all the children at last.

Yet Stanhope went through further episodes with the Joneses,

30. Edith Denegre to Stanhope Bayne-Jones, September 7, 1928, in GDC.
31. Phillips interview, 16.
32. Denegre to Chaillé, July 22, 1900, in A-24, Box 6, SBJC; Phillips interview, 20.

hard to assign a time to. During one or several summers he lived with his Aunt Mamie; she had married Julian Trist Bringier and gone to his plantation, Tezcuco, in the sugar country of south Louisiana. "Malaria, malaria, that is the cry all about," Trist's mother had written of the region, and Stanhope suffered a severe case while he lived there. But on the whole he enjoyed himself at Tezcuco. Uncle Trist was a "mythic figure," always bound for or returning from the hunt, with a shotgun on his shoulder and a brace of hounds surging about his feet. Great oaks surrounded Tezcuco, and there, among the leaves, Stanhope built himself a house where "nobody could find me."[33]

In the city, however, the old pattern of multiple parenting returned. Stanhope remembered being locked up again and "shrieking so that they could hear me all over the block, batting on the walls, trying to get out." One result may have been a lifelong disability that was almost devastating to a future scientist. An aunt would lock him into a curious prison—a long wooden stairway enclosed in a kind of chute, with doors at both ends and a single small window. She would give him a sheet of yellow paper with a column of figures and promise to let him out if he could add it up correctly. Instead, he would rush up and down the stairs, screaming and hammering on the wall. Then he would write down a number at random and thrust the paper under the door. With a rustle it would return, the sum scratched out. Distraught, he would struggle again. "Meanwhile my brother and sister would be playing out in the yard. I could see them and this little window would let the sun come through toward afternoon. I never did get that column of figures to add up."

Throughout life Stanhope couldn't add figures in a column, or keep a checkbook—"I just get the dithers." He couldn't see his own mistakes; he got telephone numbers backward; he would find "35 . . . just as valid as 53." Whether his mathematical dyslexia really came from his experiences as a child, or from some other cause, it helped to close off the universe of numbers in which the scientist must live a great part of the time. Yet the memory of his grandfather and father would drive him in a direction that he could not follow far.[34]

33. Mme. Bringier to "Browse" [Trist's brother?], August 19, 1889, in Box 2, Folder 16, JJP.
34. Phillips interview, 17–19.

His anxious childhood shaped him in other ways. This brief chronicle of his wanderings is clearly incomplete; he himself was uncertain just where he had lived and when. He had an impression of many comings and goings, impossible to comprehend. Under the pressure he learned toughness, diplomacy, and secrecy. "I think," he was to say, "this life I was leading, going from one place to the other, made me a bit secretive and [made me] want to withdraw from [people]. I think I avoided exposing myself to either criticism, or contentions, or to the opinion of strangers. I had a sort of life to myself, and I think it still continues."[35] When he spoke he was seventy-seven years old.

35. *Ibid.*, 37.

TWO

The Making of a Man

The education of the schoolboy whose friends called him Stan Jones
began in a private grammar school and a local academy. In 1902 he was
ready at thirteen to be sent away for his first experience of living and
learning among strangers. The town of Covington, north of Lake Pont-
chartrain, provided a market for local farmers and a resort for city
people oppressed by summer heat and sickness. Here too was Dixon
Academy, ruled by William A. Dixon, a friend of the Denegres. He
charged his students fifteen dollars a term for an education in the clas-
sical style.[1]

A couple of hours on the *New Camelia* steam ferryboat from New
Orleans' Milneburg Landing and a short ride on a country road took
the boy into a different world. The land was higher than the steamy
alluvium south of the lake, sandy and covered with pines; the small
rivers were spring-fed and cold, and marshy hollows lay spotted among
the low ridges of the rolling countryside.

At the academy Stan studied history and French, got "pretty far"
in Greek, and learned Latin to the point of translating Virgil. But sports
and fights were more memorable, and puberty was stirring as well. Stan
liked baseball, and he and his team's pitcher both fell in love with the
local postmistress, who was about three times the age of either. When
the pitcher, apparently an overgrown lout, made a coarse remark to the
lady, Stan challenged him.

"Did you say what I heard you had said to that lady?"

"Goddamn you, what is it to you?"

Stan was holding a *Saturday Evening Post* at the time, and he
struck the pitcher in the face with it. They agreed in best code duello
style to meet a week later on the basketball court. The outcome was
unhappy. Stan broke a knuckle on the lout's head, and with a hand out
of service got a memorable beating. Still, beatings heal; he had fulfilled

1. Brother Ephrem Hébert, *The St. Paul Story: Golden Jubilee of the Coming of the Christian Brothers to Covington, La., 1918–1968* (N.p., 1968), 4–8.

a manhood ritual that was nowhere more important than in the rural South.[2]

Even more than fights he was to remember snakes, in which the countryside was rich. Stan favored water moccasins, and took a little leather Kodak box with him into the marshes along the Bogue Falaya and Tchefuncte rivers. Finding a snake dozing on a log or suspended in a branch over a stream, he would shake it down if necessary, pin it with a forked stick behind the head, and put it into the Kodak box. Then he would bring it back to Dixon Academy and take it to the basement, a place given over to the toilets and apparently to cavernous storage spaces, and put his new pet with others he had collected. Before long he had twenty snakes, which he fed on chicks stolen from Dixon's poultry yard.

In time he expanded his operations—brought in nonpoisonous black racers, the coachwhips of Louisiana boyhood legend; cannibalistic king snakes; even a few corals, so pretty, shy, and lethal. Perhaps the snakes satisfied an appetite for risk; perhaps they reminded him of their cousins, preserved in Joseph Jones's house. But in any case, it was a lonely boy who made them his preferred company.[3]

Home for Christmas, Stan found that George and Edith had prepared a surprise gift for him—a new name. For reasons they never troubled to explain, the Denegres hyphenated him. Henceforth he was Stanhope Bayne-Jones, forever marked with the names of both his families. He returned to Dixon Academy to find his life subtly changed. He moved toward the front of the class, for seating was alphabetical. Deprived of the "comfortable mediocrity of the Js," he found himself answering more questions than ever before.

He became self-conscious about his name; he was forever having to explain it. Later, when he was an adult, problems continued. He missed callers who looked in the telephone book under J and left town without seeing him. Periodically, his bank asserted that he had no account.

In short, the name was a nuisance. But he never abandoned it and gave much evidence through a long life of finding it satisfactory. Per-

2. Phillips interview, 27.
3. *Ibid.*, 21–22.

haps its basic virtue was its truth. Was he not, in fact, the product of two clans—"a missing link," he was to say, "between two families in a feud"? Had they not now been reconciled, verbally at least, by the hyphen? Besides—Bayne-Jones: the name had flair![4]

In 1905 he was sixteen. The Denegres were thinking about his future, which must include Yale, a family tradition, where Grandfather Bayne and T. L. and Uncle Hugh had all won degrees. But could he get in? Surely something more than Dixon Academy was necessary.

Through friends, George Denegre had heard about Thacher School in California's Ojai Valley. Sherman Thacher, son of one of the most formidable conservatives of the nineteenth-century Yale faculty, had gone west as a rancher. Then he had founded a preparatory school where California boys mingled with Easterners. Informality, emphasis on sports, a great abundance of horses, and solid tutoring in subjects prominent on entrance examinations characterized the place. By the time Stan enrolled, the school had a waiting list, its own annual, *El Archivero*, school colors (orange and olive, a California medley), and organized rather than ad hoc games and sports.

The personality of the headmaster set the tone. Thacher's obsession was Purity, his touchstone word, and in regard to sex he meant exactly that. On the other hand, discipline was enlightened, maintained largely by Thacher's benevolence and firmness. He was said to have struck a boy only once, a well-merited reaction to a practical joke. The school was expensive and projected an image of all the Progressive Era held dear—manliness, virtue, good sense, and rapid advancement—in this case, to a prestigious university.[5]

Stan's departure was nerve-wracking. A yellow fever epidemic was raging in New Orleans. For the first time the city was able to fight back, using methods that Stan's second cousin, Col. William C. Gorgas, had devised to conquer the disease in Havana. But the city's neighbors were taking no chances. Traditionally, "shotgun quarantines" excluded New

4. *Ibid.*, 24–25.
5. LeRoy McKim Makepeace, *Sherman Thacher and His School* (New Haven, 1941), 7, 70, 87, 104–105, 149, 151.

Orleans people, goods, and even mail during an epidemic. To try to avoid being turned back, Stan appeared before a doctor of the Public Health and Marine Hospital Service and received a certificate that he was free from symptoms. He carried the document with him when he left for California on September 4. Nevertheless, the Texas border had been closed, and mobs there stoned and shot at trains from Louisiana. The doors of Stan's coach were nailed shut and screens tacked over the windows, and he reached California by way of Chicago and Santa Fe.[6]

After the harrowing trip, he was received cordially. By all evidence he was a success at Thacher School. He was away from his families and the stresses associated with them, secure in a kind of society he now knew well. The horses were welcome, the sports congenial, and he had learned somewhere to play the guitar. He gave clear signs of developing a persona that was to serve him well—an easy geniality that had the double purpose of drawing people to him while keeping them a certain distance away. Belonging nowhere, he began to learn how to be welcome everywhere, an art that demands ready warmth and inner reserve.

In his year in the Ojai Valley he took second honors in algebra, first in Greek composition. He studied Cicero, placed second in English, and made the headmaster's list for freedom from discreditable marks for lateness, misconduct, and untidiness. He served as an upperclass prefect and a member of the Outdoor Committee. (Was this the great committeeman's first?) He won the Gymkhana that December. His nickname at the school was Jonah, and unlike his namesake, he was popular. His guitar was a feature of the school, and he played "sentimental rag-time" in his room. "'Come and listen to the music' is our only advice," said *El Archivero*.[7]

During his second term (the school year was divided into three) a new student moved into the next room. Andrew Dickson White was the grandson and namesake of the cofounder and president of Cornell University. He came from a well-to-do family in Syracuse, New York, a bustling railroad town embellished with a Hamilton S. White monu-

6. Certificate in A-26, Box 6, SBJC; see also Phillips interview, 330.

7. *El Archivero, 1906: The Ninth Volume of the Thacher School Annual* (Nordhoff, Calif., 1906), 39, 47, 72–73, 79, 87, 89, in A-28, Box 6, SBJC.

ment and a White Memorial Building. Stan was duly impressed. White was "a highly cultivated and educated young fellow. . . . How he happened to find something congenial in me was astonishing to me because we were very different."[8]

Perhaps White sensed that both had found youth difficult. Apparently, they traded painful memories. Besides likeness as an attraction, there was unlikeness: Stanhope was almost out of his own time of confusion while White, far more troubled, was sinking deeper into his, driven, perhaps (though his letters are ambiguous), by a homosexual inclination he could not tolerate in himself—in a *White*.

In any case, a dependent character found a strong one, a lonely boy a friend. "The three short months after you became 'Jonah' to me . . . were the happiest and the greatest I have ever known," White wrote. "I hate this mushy sort of talk, but I wanted you to know that there is no one in the world whom I have felt for as I have for you. I want you to know it, for I must sooner or later lose the power of telling you—and it may be sooner, for such is often 'The course of human events.' Ever faithfully, A."[9]

Stan graduated from Thacher on June 12, 1906, and went traveling. A lively summer took him from Bronxville, New York, where Uncle Hugh now resided, to Biloxi, where Tante E still kept Malua. The year just past had been important, for he had gone among strangers and succeeded.

But White, home in Syracuse, brooded about death, which more and more seemed to him the cure-all for life's tangles. He sent Jonah a postcard view of the entrance to Oakwood Cemetery, and on the back again quoted the Declaration of Independence—"When in the course of human events it becomes necessary." In January, 1907, back at Thacher, he made a will, leaving Jonah his horse, Rush, and "what little personal property I possess."[10]

He could not wait to be gone. On the last day of January he took part in the usual morning calisthenics. He admitted to Thacher that he

8. Phillips interview, 38.
9. Andrew Dickson White to Bayne-Jones, November 15, 1906, January 18, 1907, and *El Archivero*, 39, all in A-28, Box 6, SBJC.
10. Items in A-28, Box 6, SBJC.

had been feeling a little depressed lately but joked that it was only indigestion, after all. He exchanged another joke with the housemother of his building, then went to his room. There he took a .22 caliber revolver from his trunk and shot himself through the roof of the mouth.

In a letter to White's family, Thacher wrote that the boy's marks were high, he had no disciplinary problems, his relations with both boys and teachers were "particularly good," and his health was excellent. Nevertheless, the idea of suicide had evidently been in his mind for years; he had kept the revolver, against the rules, locked in his trunk for the time when he would use it. He had spoken of his intentions to "an intimate friend or two, who did not however, believe him to be entirely serious." Thacher left the Ojai Valley to accompany the body home.[11]

Stan wrote to the bereaved family, offering condolences, and they had heard of him: Andrew's uncle wrote back that the dead boy had "esteemed you as his best friend, and regarded you also as an example." Andrew's mother, Anne Bruce White, invited him to visit and fell as easily under his burgeoning charm as her son had. "I can see why my beautiful boy loved you . . . remember my adopted affection for you."[12]

And here the biographer meets a difficult problem. Did Andrew's mother become Stan's lover? It seems certain, on the basis of contemporary references, that—perhaps now, perhaps while he was a student at Yale—he became involved in a lengthy affair with an older woman. Tante E, who knew the facts of the matter, wrote that her nephew was drawn by "generous & kindly sympathy & pity for a stricken mother" into a liaison that lasted "a long time." Certainly Stan's visits to the Whites were many, and continued over the years of college and medical school in a way that suggests some central attraction. But the evidence is at best uncertain.[13]

Better documented was his admiration for Andrew's distinguished

11. *The Ojai* (Nordhoff, Calif.), February 9, 1907.
12. Dwight H. Bruce to Bayne-Jones, February 14, 1907, and Anne Bruce White to Bayne Jones, [n.d.], both in A-28, Box 6, SBJC.
13. Tante E. to Bayne-Jones, July 27, 1928, in GDC.

grandfather. Until this time, Stan's religion had faithfully reflected his raising. Baptized a Catholic, in Minna's faith, he collided with the varied beliefs of his other relatives as he lived with each in turn. At Joseph Jones's house, news of the death of John Calvin had not been received, and the word of the doctor's brother-in-law, a Presbyterian clergyman, ruled. Aunt Susie Jones was more interested in her mother's Episcopal faith; when Stan lived with her, he went to St. Paul's and sang for a time in the choir, until he was exiled for fighting.

Meanwhile, the Denegres brought up his brother and sister as Catholics, and Stan, too, returned to that communion when he joined them. But the Denegres' Catholicism was liberal, casual about the regulations of Church or diocese. (As became a lawyer, George discovered that a medieval pope had declared duck to be a form of fish, and so the family ate duck on Fridays when they pleased.) Dixon and Thacher schools both had routine prayers, which the students attended while thinking of something else.[14]

The conclusion that Stan drew from his mixed upbringing was that a "great difference [existed] between what I later learned to call religion as distinct from theology." Necessarily, he learned early to distinguish between the impulse toward religion and its institutional forms, between faith and dogma, between reverence and piety. He soon read—may, under Andrew White's encouragement, already have read—President White's "very satisfying, huge, two volume treatise" called *A History of the Warfare of Science with Theology*. White attacked superstition and clericalism. Science would gradually improve religion, he believed, by ridding it of the time-worn forms of sacerdotalism that encumbered it. The purified end result would be the recognition of "'a Power in the universe, not ourselves, which makes for righteousness,' and . . . the love of God and of our neighbor."[15]

This deism became in Stan's mind something simpler. He attained—it is hard to say when—"a respect for something, though I don't know what it is." As an adult he did not believe in anything he chose to call God, or in a life after death, or in the improbabilities of

14. Phillips interview, 30–33.
15. *Ibid.*, 30, 32; Andrew Dickson White, *A History of the Warfare of Science with Theology* (1896; rpr. New York, 1960), xii.

the creed he had recited in so many different formats. He became much like W. Somerset Maugham's archetypal Unitarian, who disbelieved very earnestly almost everything that everyone else believed, yet kept a firm sustaining faith in he did not quite know what. Perhaps Stan would have agreed with his contemporary, the professionally skeptical H. L. Mencken, whom he later met in Baltimore. Religion, wrote Mencken in 1916, is debased by the pretense of knowing the unknowable, and the most "satisfying and ecstatic faith" is one which "trusts absolutely without professing to know at all."[16]

For Stan a similar viewpoint grew out of his extraordinary relationship with the Whites. In one family he found a friend, a prophet, and perhaps a lover. The friendship was brief and ended in death; the sexual relationship was long but ran its course in time. The attitude of reverent unbelief lasted through his lifetime, the most durable monument to the year when he was seventeen and lived in the Ojai Valley.

Stan entered Yale feeling that he was a country mouse among the city mice. Yet he had tasted success at Thacher and was resolved to win more. He wanted not merely to pass Yale but to make a nobody—himself—into a somebody.

He had certain advantages. Emotionally, he was older than his years. Willful as only one can be whose wishes have been much thwarted, he had also learned in a long succession of foster homes and two boarding schools that survival demanded constant diplomacy. He had been obliged to watch people, to try to anticipate their reactions, and he knew how to fight when he had to, with his fists or without.

But none of that sufficed in the Ivy League. Shortly after he arrived at Yale, Stan was measured at the gym and put through a series of standard tests, which revealed only that he was a youth of middle height, lightly built, moderately athletic. There was nothing in his classwork to set him apart from the run of ordinary, fairly bright undergraduates. His appearance did nothing to dispel the impression of

16. Phillips interview, 34; Alistair Cooke, ed., *The Vintage Mencken* (New York, n.d.), 69; Maugham, *Of Human Bondage* (New York, 1942), 135.

ordinariness. He had straw-colored hair and a bit of a New Orleans accent, pronouncing his native city N'Awleeuns. His family was well-to-do but far from rich. Thacher School was all very well, but it won him no notice among the graduates of prestigious prep schools, all of whom seemed to know one another. The perpetual outsider wanted desperately to be an insider. Instead, he would "walk around the streets and look at the lighted windows and hear people laugh," but he himself had "nothing to laugh about."[17]

Then the campus paper offered him a ladder to climb on. The Yale *Daily News* had been launched to convey the "latest news, and short, pithy articles of interest." Editorial posts automatically made their possessors persons of significance on campus, and—what must have caught Stan's eye—they were won by pure competition. Hopefuls were obliged to "heel," to get copy for the paper. Whoever submitted the most published words won the job. That became Stan's goal.

He found it "very, very strenuous," because news had to be pursued in the evening, after a day in class. As the name implied, heeling usually involved considerable expense of shoe leather. Each competition lasted half a year, and Stan went through three of them before he won with 67,475 words to his nearest competitor's 66,800. It was a struggle, and he had paid a price—a grade average in the 250 range against a possible 400. But the victory was intensely sweet.[18]

Perhaps success is its own reward. By all indications, Stan's life flowered during his last two years at Yale. He found a congenial roommate in a midwesterner, Howard Vincent O'Brien, inevitably known as Pat. They lived together "under the eaves of Durfee Hall," forming a friendship that lasted until O'Brien's death in 1947. To their later, perhaps rosy recollections, they shared their money and had not a single serious quarrel. Their days began when a bell chimed at 8 A.M. announcing compulsory chapel, rousing them to light the gas mantle and scurry down three flights of stairs to wash. A horde of students, responding to the "theological alarm clock," tumbled outside, in wet

17. Test papers and measurements in A-30, Box 7, SBJC; see also Phillips interview, 39–40.
18. Dean's warning, January 7, 1908, and Sherman Thacher to Bayne-Jones, April 15, 1908, in A-30, Box 7, SBJC; Phillips interview, 40–41.

weather pulling galoshes over bare feet and throwing raincoats over pajamas.

Classes shared time with the immemorial interests of student life. A woman walking across the all-male campus drew watchers to the windows, warned by a cry of "Fire!" from whomever spotted her first. Students drank delicious cream ale in Tuttle's, "that dark hole"; they studied the mysteries of pool in a hall with curtained windows; they attended the Grand Theater, where for a quarter they could "hiss the villainies of Nelly the Cloak Model's betrayer"; they took their clothes to Rosie the suit-presser, "whose cheer no vicissitudes could alter." When low in funds, they borrowed money from a local dealer in wood and old clothes. Inevitably, they experimented with drunkenness, Pat on occasion "going to bed in the fireplace."[19]

With his Uncle Hugh Bayne, Stan explored the theaters of New Haven. He had invitations to dinner and to cards; he filled his program at dances; he was elected by the junior class a member of the promenade committee; he became president of the freshman athletic committee and got the sweet taste of being an upperclassman guiding the young. Remarkably, his grades improved, rising to a 330 or 340 average. In no sense did he dazzle Yale by his brilliance, but he did something that must have been infinitely more satisfying. Against all odds he was a success, a Zeta Tau, a fairly big man on campus.

He even spent Christmas 1909 at the White House, by courtesy of Uncle Hugh, one of whose associates at his Wall Street law firm was Henry W. Taft, the president's brother. In those days the First Family was genuinely that and no more: as Stan wrote to Tante E, "there is a family like any other family in this house." An invitation from them was a signal honor but not a summons into a semiroyal presence, and Stan slept in Lincoln's bedroom like a visiting potentate.

One result of the visit was a closer acquaintance with the president's son, Robert. A classmate at Yale, the future senator and Republican candidate for president was one of those young men from a prestigious background who had at first been unknown and unknowable to

19. Boston *Globe*, March 21, 1936; Howard Vincent O'Brien, "All Things Considered," Chicago *Daily News*, January 30, 1942; Bayne-Jones to O'Brien, July 31, 1933, in A-32, Box 7, SBJC.

Stan. Not only privilege but ability marked him off: he was a prize-winning scholar, a mathematician, an accomplished debater, while Stan was a middling student at best, heeling for the paper. The awesome figure of the campus turned out to be quite another man at home. The mood of the mansion was relaxed and festive; the vast figure of the chief executive was a good approximation of Father Christmas; the guests played games, turning out the lights for hide-and-seek; Stan rode horseback with the Tafts in Rock Creek Park, a snowy semi-wilderness laced with trails. Throughout, he saw a side of Robert A. Taft that would have seemed remarkable to Americans who later knew only a granitic public image: "He was gay but restrained . . . a charming person, very thoughtful, rather full of fun."[20] Here too was the basis for a friendship that lasted a lifetime.

The ultimate accolade, shared with Taft, came at the end of Stan's junior year. As usual on Tap Day, the students gathered while representatives of the senior societies passed among them. In perfect confidence Stanhope waited under a tree, and sure enough he felt a touch on his shoulder, and a voice said, "Go to your room." There a committee of men from Skull and Bones arrived to tender him the offer of membership.[21] He did not decline.

Some troubles, of course, do not yield to charm or even to success. A letter from his sister Marian reached him at Durfee Hall in February, 1909, and revived the past in a particularly acute way.

"With some of the facts of your letter I was familiar," he replied, in the cautious, objective style he had already adopted, "but of the manner of my father's death—suicide—I knew nothing." He took a refuge that was to become customary with him: "My nature may be shallow—but painful considerations do not remain with me long." He

20. Bayne-Jones to Tante E (Edith Bayne Denegre), Christmas Day, [1909], in A-28, Box 6, SBJC; Stanhope Bayne-Jones, interview with Harry K. Jeffrey, August 28, 1967, Washington, D.C., in Senator Robert A. Taft Project, Oral History Research Office, Columbia University, New York, N.Y. Bayne-Jones, then an old man, recalled that Robert Taft had invited him to the White House but could not recall why; contemporary references support the version in the text.

21. Phillips interview, 45; Brooks Mather Kelley, Yale: A History (New Haven, 1974), 223–26; Loomis Havemeyer, "Go to Your Room" : A Story of Undergraduate Societies and Fraternities at Yale (New Haven, 1960), 48–72.

regretted the suffering that the news, wherever she learned it, had caused her. He drew a significant comparison: "There is in my class the son of Morse, the New York banker who is now in the penitentiary. This fact has never had the least conscious effect—except for sympathy—upon my relations with that classmate, and I apply the same thing to myself. As I said, I don't judge my father—and the sense of no responsibility prevents a great deal of the pain you speak of. . . . At times I think of it completely dispassionately."[22]

His life was taking shape, and his choice of a profession furthered the process. "I never had any doubts and I never had any agony such as some of my classmates at Yale had," he would say later. "For me it was all settled by the stars long ago." For him, medicine was the inevitable calling.[23]

He knew also where he wanted to study: Johns Hopkins in Baltimore. His choice reflected old associations, family themes. Minna Bayne had attended a Catholic school in Maryland; the family had developed a habit of staying in Baltimore when they visited her, and the friendships they had formed there lingered, bringing the Denegres back to the city on the Chesapeake long after her death. Tante E knew William Sydney Thayer, a man of considerable distinction and charm who was a professor of medicine at Hopkins. Stan himself, going and returning to Yale, often admired the dome and staring brick towers of the hospital.[24]

He may not yet have been aware of other, more solid reasons for favoring Johns Hopkins. In 1910, the year of his graduation from Yale, Abraham Flexner published a report commissioned by the Carnegie Foundation for the Advancement of Learning that left little doubt why an ambitious young man should want to study there. Customarily abrasive, Flexner was moved almost to lyricism by the Baltimore school. It was, he wrote, one of the best, if not absolutely the best, in the country. It required for entrance a college degree that included satisfactory work

22. Bayne-Jones to Marian Jones, February 14, 1909, in A-28, Box 6, SBJC.
23. Phillips interview, 15.
24. Ibid., 55–57.

in the three fundamental sciences—chemistry, physics, and biology. The entrant must also be able to read French and German, giving him access to the medical literature of Europe. The school's laboratories were "in every aspect unexcelled," its clinical facilities "practically ideal."[25]

Perhaps Stan chose the right school for the wrong reasons; perhaps a deep-laid drive toward the best and highest was already at work in him. In either case, he seemed to have little chance of attending Hopkins, for Tante E had decided that he belonged at home. His brother was to enter Yale; his sister had married and moved out of the Denegre house. Marian had not gone far—in fact, she lived across the street, which was not even a wide one. But she no longer belonged to Tante E as in the past. Redoubtable Edith was left alone with George and a white poodle she had bought and named Bouche Troue—in the fractured French of the city, "Stopgap." The dog failed to live up to its name. When Stan pleaded for Johns Hopkins, Edith replied that she and Uncle George were lonely and that "you'd better come home." He surrendered to her wishes; most people did.[26]

New Orleans' best medical education was offered by Tulane University, and undeniably it was something of a comedown. Far from the bottom of American medical schools, Tulane was also a long way from the top. Flexner, himself a Kentuckian, recognized the poverty of the South, saw Tulane in its regional context, and was unwontedly kind: "The medical department of Tulane University is one of the very few existing southern schools that deserve development," he judged. Its library was small, but its laboratories were new and excellent, and its students learned the clinician's art at the patient's bedside in Charity Hospital, a facility then of 1,050 beds. But Tulane could not be compared to Johns Hopkins. It accepted a high-school certificate for admission; its endowment was less than $1 million as against Hopkins' $3.6 million; it was a school of promise, a regional leader—but no more.[27]

With his Yale degree in hand, Stan must have known that he

25. Abraham Flexner, *Medical Education in the United States and Canada: A Report to the Carnegie Foundation for the Advancement of Teaching* (New York, 1972), 28, 30.
26. Phillips interview, 49.
27. Flexner, *Medical Education*, 233.

was qualified to attempt the best. In his later years at Yale he had gone from purely literary studies to a mixed regime of science and liberal arts that was coming to characterize much of American higher education. Fascinated though he was by lectures on Samuel Johnson and the eighteenth-century world, and on modern dramatists such as Shaw and Pinero, Stan had also developed a liking for chemistry. He had progressed far enough to be accepted as a student by Yale's physiological chemist, Russell Chittenden. An old house in New Haven had been converted into the Sheffield Scientific School, and Sheffield—with its lively and critical dean, its dismal labs, its crowds of students eager to "wipe the eye" of Yale conservatives—had been an exciting place. Even the smells and hard work had agreed with Stan: Were they not parts of his grandfather's world? The milieu was too much like the house of old Dr. Jones not to please. He had discovered in the laboratory a workshop and refuge that was to claim a great part of his life.[28]

He had the necessary degree, an introductory knowledge of one basic science, a fair command of French, and a reading knowledge of German. But he did not have Hopkins. His unhappy transition to Tulane Medical School took place in the fall of 1910. Students spent their first two years studying anatomy and the basic sciences in the new graystone Richardson Memorial building on the pleasant Uptown campus, some thirty blocks from the Denegre house by the electric trolley. Examinations had become rigorous and frequent. Some members of the faculty—notably the vascular surgeon Rudolph Matas, the malariologist Charles C. Bass, and dean Isador Dyer, a founder of the Carville hospital for lepers—had won national or international renown.

But Stan saw his fellow students with jaundiced eyes. Thirty years before, a president of Harvard had complained that "an American physician or surgeon may be, and often is, a coarse and uncultivated person."[29] If Stan's recollections can be trusted, this tradition lingered at Tulane in the year of the Flexner Report. The university did not require

28. Phillips interview, 47–49. The best overview of medical education at the time is to be found in Kenneth M. Ludmerer, *Learning to Heal: The Development of American Medical Education* (New York, 1985), especially 6, 167.

29. John Duffy, *The Tulane University Medical Center: One Hundred and Fifty Years of Medical Education* (Baton Rouge, 1984), 90, 94, 107, 118, 123, 127; Ludmerer, *Learning to Heal*, 13.

even two years of college work as a prerequisite for entrance—a standard that, when adopted, would give a great advantage to young people of the middle and upper classes. But in 1910 many of the students apparently were country boys with very little education at all.

Stan found them rough company for meeting the shock of gross anatomy. The dead house stank as usual of formalin and human flesh in a state of semi-arrested decay. Teamed with a Georgia youth, Stan tried to work out "all the muscles and nerves very carefully." Meanwhile, the Georgian took a knife to the buttocks of the cadaver and "cut one side . . . off like a ham and took it to the professor. He was finished with his dissection in five minutes."[30]

Despite the hint of snobbery, Stan was as usual popular, becoming president of his class. But there was no denying that a good deal of adaptability was needed to handle his classmates. Abraham Louis Metz, a chemistry teacher, stayed in his memory as a man who had found a way to reach the country boys. Chalking *Na* on the blackboard, he said, "Here's Mr. Sodium. He's blond and debonair, and he's walking down the beach." Up went *Cl*. "This is Miss Chlorine, and she's green-eyed and avid." Then, writing *NaCl*, the formula for common salt, he demanded, "Name their baby!"

Stan found himself in several predicaments when backwoods democracy collided with the authoritarian demands of learning. As class president, he was deputized by his fellow students to ask the Tulane trustees to eliminate the neurology course that, as taught by a strict professor, they thought had been added to the curriculum merely to spite them. On another occasion, he claimed many years later, he received word that the students had haled an unpopular teacher down to the levee and stripped him as the first step toward tarring and feathering him. Stan had to rush down to stop the exercise before it reached its painful conclusion.

But his memories of Tulane were not all negative. Of Metz's unorthodox methods he said later, "That's a good way to teach." And it was Metz who enticed him into his first piece of real research, an attempt to synthesize tryptophane, an amino acid, from one of the con-

---

30. Phillips interview, 50.

stituents of milk. The attempt was unsuccessful, as Metz had predicted it would be, but the effort lingered in his pupil's memory.[31]

On the financial side, Tulane had distinct advantages: because Joseph Jones had been a professor there, Stan received a scholarship. His inheritance was not large—apparently about $19,000 at the turn of the century. Its sources were his share of Minna's estate, a second legacy left by an aunt in Georgia, and a small share in Joseph Jones's estate that was bought out by the widow. As managed by George Denegre, the estate brought in about $1,000 a year. Doled out to Stan at $83.33 a month, the money had paid his basic expenses—food, shelter, probably some part of his clothing—through his years at Thacher and Yale. Because Thacher was accounted an expensive school, and Yale tuition amounted to $400 a year, it could hardly have paid for everything. In old age, Stan, though inclined to exaggerate what a dollar could buy in his youth, admitted that the sources of his income were not clear: "I don't know who put the money up, to tell you the truth."

The most logical candidates were the Denegres, and it could only have been with their assent that Stan, after one year at Tulane, was able to resume his quest for a Johns Hopkins medical degree.[32]

Stan must have been poor company for Tante E. He lived in the attic of the Denegre house, in a room with a single bed. He avoided dances, if he could, and stayed away from the Mardi Gras festivities of 1911. Perhaps he was changing; medicine was demanding, and his interest was caught as his father's and his grandfather's had been. Or was his new-found dourness a way of communicating his unhappiness?

In any case, by the end of the school year the Denegres were ready to see him go. Stan had been reading Emerson, finding in the essay on self-reliance the sage's typical belief that one should leave a house in which one is not happy, rather than endure and try to make a go of it. One evening about nine o'clock he walked downstairs, in great trepidation, to the library where George and Edith sat in facing chairs,

31. *Ibid.*, 51.
32. *Ibid.*, 50.

reading. Expecting trouble, he told them that he wanted to go. With the customary amazement of youth, unable to believe that its elders find it as trying as it finds them, he heard them agree at once. "We were all together in no time."[33]

Now he sat down and wrote possibly the most important letters of his life: carefully crafted appeals to Johns Hopkins professors William H. Welch and W. H. Howell to admit him to the second year class, provided he made up first-year courses that were given there but not at Tulane. Howell's agreement, and especially Welch's, Stan considered "one of the achievements of anybody in the world." For in approaching Welch he had taken his first step toward the man who, more than any other, was the teacher not only of medical students but of American medicine.

Howell suggested either Chicago or Ann Arbor for the summer courses Stan needed in physiology and bacteriology. Choosing Rush Medical College in Chicago, Stan traveled to the big midwestern city and spent the hot months in another of those roosts the migratory student learns to inhabit. He studied physiology with Ajax Carlson—a large, loud, opinionated man who was a Pied Piper among the students because of his perfect lack of pretense. Bacteriology was taught routinely and adequately. Informed but uninspired, Stan felt as yet no urge to make the study of microscopic life a specialty of his own.[34]

Away from home, with only two courses and much free time, he may have devoted his most serious thinking to a subject far removed from medicine. Just prior to his move to Chicago, he had explored Ithaca as the guest of Andrew Dickson White. The Cornell president showed him the campus he had built and discussed the great issues of the day with him, including the perennially burning Negro Question. White had found Cornell's few blacks to be "pretty good students," and he suggested, somewhat naïvely, that the South disfranchise the ignorant by setting high educational qualifications for voting. "By strict ap-

33. *Ibid.*, 53.
34. *Ibid.*, 57, 60–61; Diary of Stanhope Bayne-Jones, 1911, in A-28, Box 6, SBJC; Bayne-Jones to Welch, with Welch's marginal comments, February 12, 1911, in GDC. On Welch, see Hans Zinsser, *As I Remember Him: The Biography of R.S.* (Boston, 1940), 110, and citations in Chapter Three below.

plication of such a standard," he suggested, "you can *constitutionally* get rid of nearly all your negro vote and a large percentage of an ignorant white vote and at the same time do something that this country badly needs—raise the right of suffrage to a respected plane."

Stan knew better than to believe this tory wisdom. The triumph of Jim Crow in the region had taken place largely during the past ten years, and he knew that disfranchisement had to do with power, not education. To White he quoted George Denegre's candid view that blacks ought to be kept from voting legally if possible and by force if necessary, in order to prevent them from becoming the region's balance of power. To this, White replied firmly that forcible repression could never be just, a declaration, coming from a "venerable, majestic . . . most magnetic . . . grand old man," that made a deep impression on Stan.[35]

He continued to think it over in Chicago. A visit to the library led him by accident to a shelf of books about the Negro, and that in turn to further mulling of the questions of race, power, and justice. The subject still preoccupied him at the end of the year, when he was once again invited to the White House, this time by Robert Taft.

For the third time William Howard Taft presided at Christmas in the executive mansion. Dinner on Christmas Eve passed in silence, the president applying more attention to "what went into his mouth than what came out of it." Stan had hoped for "improvement" by listening to presidential wisdom, but those formidable jaws were otherwise engaged.

The evening was again, as in 1909, a tableau—the president leading the recitation of "The Night Before Christmas," a fire burning in the Red Room, a potted holly tree catching the gleams with its polished red berries. To Stan the electric lights in the bronze chandelier overhead seemed somehow less noticeable (because less in tune) than the old Monroe candlesticks standing before a tall mirror. On Christmas Day, after church, he found his quarry more vulnerable and boldly asked the chief executive about the Negro Question.

This time he got the enlightenment he sought. Taft declared that

35. Diary, 1911, in A-28, Box 6, SBJC.

he appointed Negroes to office "in places where he found them worthy and the sentiment of the community was not against them" and went on to mock the racial fears that sustained the one-party system in the South. Thinking it over, Stan concluded that black officeholders, merely by carrying out responsible tasks, demolished the assumption of racial inferiority that was the only possible justification for their race's exclusion.

"To me," he wrote, "the positions gained by these men are striking proof of what the race may become in freedom rather than the animal-like creature . . . in the South, where neglect and suppression perpetuate his brutishness." Typically, this freethinking young conservative reached a liberal position on the basis of jobs done, positions attained. In so doing he began to separate himself from the worst aspect of a heritage to which, in other matters, he would remain devoted. If education means more than schooling, Stan's achievements in 1911 went beyond his courses at Chicago, or even his entry into Hopkins.[36]

Yet he still had something of the schoolboy's habit of leisurely summers and almost missed the whole point of his summer's work at Rush. Early in August he took another brief trip to Syracuse to visit Anne Bruce White, returning to Chicago in time for his examinations. In September, the term over and his courses passed, he lingered there, reading for his own pleasure. Suddenly he realized that the day set for his meeting with the admissions committee at Hopkins had passed.

He caught a train to Baltimore, and appeared alone in the dean's office, the only candidate for admission whose fate was still to be decided. The committee assembled to confront the latecomer under its chairman, J. Whitridge Williams, professor of obstetrics, a huge man known as "Bull." With him were William Welch, W. H. Howell, and Franklin P. Mall, the anatomist. Stan walked in, holding his derby hat in hand.

Someone said, "Won't you have a seat?" Stan carefully put his hat on an empty chair and sat down on it.

36. *Ibid.*

With infinite tact, all members of the committee managed to act as if he had not done what he had done. Instead of the grilling he expected, they conversed quietly with him; that was the aim of the exercise, to get a feeling for the candidate. Slowly, because everyone else was acting normally, he began to do so, too. At the end of the meeting, Mall—Stan was later to learn that this tall, intelligent man had a gift for saying "sharp things in a gentle manner"—remarked:

"You can get up off your hat now. That's not a sacrifice demanded of the neophyte here."

Stan had been accepted at Hopkins.[37]

37. Phillips interview, 58, 69. The story sounds almost too good to be true, but Bayne-Jones insisted it was the truth and had not altogether recovered from his embarrassment fifty-five years later.

THREE

The Making of a Doctor

The Baltimore of those times is hard to see nowadays except through the eyes of its great journalist, H. L. Mencken. Like Stan's native New Orleans, Baltimore was a middle-sized seaport, conventionally wicked. Much given to the pleasures of the table, it drew the raw material of its feasts from what Mencken called the "immense protein factory" of Chesapeake Bay. Though the city benefited from its location near the national centers of the East Coast, Baltimore was nonetheless defensive, well aware that it lacked Washington's power, Philadelphia's history, Boston's culture, and New York's metropolitan status.

It was all the prouder of what it did have—especially its new university. Like any college town, Baltimore excepted from its general ban on outsiders those who were associated with Johns Hopkins. Its medical practitioners, thirty years earlier resentful and suspicious of the men and ideas brought by the faculty, had grown accustomed to their city's role as something like a capital of American medicine.[1]

In this unfamiliar city of smoky red brick and gothic pastiche, Stan sought a place to live. By what precise process he could not later remember, but with an instinct that was to serve him well, he made his way to the rowhouse on St. Paul Street where William Welch—"a very big, portly man with a very large abdominal section, very handsome, dignified, pleasant-voiced, kindly"—occupied bachelor quarters. Stan secured a room directly above Welch's bedroom and, by his later admission, moved his bed over the doctor's, in order to absorb any radiations of genius that might ascend in the night.[2]

The drive toward prominence that had drawn him to White at school and to Taft in college was at work again. No mere toady, Stan

---

1. Alistair Cooke, ed., *The Vintage Mencken* (New York, 1955), 5; Simon Flexner and James Thomas Flexner, *William Henry Welch and the Heroic Age of American Medicine* (1941, New York; rpr., 1966), 153–56, and Donald Fleming, *William H. Welch and the Rise of Modern Medicine* (Boston, 1954), 79.

2. Phillips interview, 63, 66, 68.

approached his betters in order to win their respect as well as their indulgence. But he unquestionably felt the need of the perennial outsider to draw close to sources of power. For too long, others had made decisions behind closed doors that shaped his life. He wanted to get behind those doors, to find out what was going on and to make some of the decisions himself. More poignant was his need to find some powerful older man to occupy his father's vacant niche. Welch—"Popsy" to all his students—was, for the time being, elected.

There were surprising similarities between the sixty-four-year-old, New England-born professor and the twenty-two-year-old student in the room above. Welch, like Stan, had lost his mother while still young. He too had attended Yale, had been tapped for Skull and Bones, and had entered the profession of medicine that was his father's occupation—indeed, his father's life. Now a fixture of Johns Hopkins, Welch lived to the full the life of the American academic physician that he had done much to define. He had also become, by election, a Baltimorean. He was a fan of the Orioles, a *bon vivant* who loved to give elegant dinners at the Maryland Club, where he introduced his students, accustomed to poor fare, to the "diamond-backed terrapin, wild duck, pearly soft-shelled crabs, and . . . the prodigious oysters of [the Chesapeake's] teeming waters."

The students worshiped him, for he treated them as colleagues, but they did not draw too close, for reserve as much as cordiality marked Welch as a teacher. His tact was legendary. Stan was often to tell the story of how Mary Simmons, their landlady, answered the doctor's ring at the bell one night, with harsh words ready for a boarder who had forgotten his key. But Welch came armed with the floral centerpiece of the dinner party he had attended; he piled it into her arms and slipped upstairs to bed unscolded.[3]

Welch was a pillar of the new medical education; he had launched and edited for a time the nation's first journal of experimental medicine; he advised university presidents and made the careers of the promising young. He entertained visiting celebrities, carefully preparing himself in advance to talk on matters that would interest them. He knew Fred-

3. Flexner and Flexner, *William Henry Welch*, 168.

erick T. Gates, the Baptist preacher who was guiding part of the Rocke-feller fortune into medical channels. Through Gates, Welch had be-come the disburser of the first Rockefeller grants for medical research. In 1906 he had been made a trustee of the Carnegie Institution as well. In this, too, Welch was a leader: foundation money was the first key to bringing American medical research into contention as a world force. Welch was more than a charming pedagogue. He had a sense of present and future power in the medical world.[4]

Increasingly, the world of the medical practitioner was diverging from that of the teacher and the researcher. During the nineteenth century, many powerful doctors had practiced a specialty while teach-ing in medical schools of which they were part owners. But salaried academics had helped to shape medical school reform, lately gaining a new and powerful voice through the Council on Medical Education of the recently reorganized American Medical Association. With the growth of clinical research, the researcher-teacher and the practitioner, each necessary to the other, would find a point of union in the clinical scientist who worked at the patient's bedside in a teaching hospital, of which Hopkins was a model.

Yet two distinct roads were opening in American medicine. In the friendly atmosphere of the Progressive Era, devoted to centralization and science and reform, the AMA developed as the acknowledged voice of the profession, backing reforms that interested doctors and organiz-ing its members as a national force. In its political role it emerged as an increasingly powerful pressure group dominated by specialists, voicing the ideology of the traditional successful practitioner. Welch spoke for quite another kind of physician—salaried in full or in part, his work subsidized and oriented toward the laboratory and the clinic. As prac-titioners lost control of medical education, the medical schools drew closer to the universities, of which increasingly they formed a part. This was the world that Stan was entering; that it would absorb a great part of his life, no one could yet have guessed.[5]

4. Phillips interview, 64–65; Flexner and Flexner, *William Henry Welch*, 269–78, 292.
5. John Duffy, *The Healers: A History of American Medicine* (1976; rpr. Urbana, Ill., 1979), 313; Paul Starr, *The Social Transformation of American Medicine* (New York, 1982), 121–23; Oliver Garceau, *The Political Life of the American Medical Association* (Hamden, Conn., 1961), 54–55, 57.

Stan began his studies at a time when the new scientific medicine, though firmly established, had not yet overwhelmed the ancient liberal art. For a brief time, a medical education was almost a course in universalism. Like other students, Stan had begun by immersing himself in the literary culture of the West. Now he would spend years learning to combine the discipline of the laboratory with the enforced human contact of the hospital and the examining room. Medicine, said one of his teachers, compelled the thoughtful student to master habits of hard work and a "considered correlation of the fundamental sciences," even as it brought him face to face with "the misery, the courage and cowardice, of his fellow creatures."[6]

Science had revolutionized medicine, and each discovery seemed to promise others. In the mid-nineteenth century, European studies of economically important problems—fermentation, silkworm disease, anthrax—had gradually rehabilitated an old belief that minute living creatures caused some forms of illness. Meanwhile, a few medical scientists had arrived at the insight that each disease is specific, a single entity with a unique cause. The cellular basis of life was established. Beginning with the demonstration in 1876 by the German experimenter Robert Koch that a spore- forming, rod-shaped bacillus was the cause of anthrax, one major disease after another was shown to have a specific microbial cause.

Since then, the work of the pioneers of the germ theory had been steadily amplified and extended. Further light on the transmission of disease had come through the discovery that vectors—carriers or intermediate hosts—can transmit the organisms that cause disease. As a result, the fifty-year-old struggle of doctors, statisticians, and engineers to improve public health through preventive medicine found new weapons and new heroes. (Few were more celebrated than Stan's second cousin, "Uncle Willy" Gorgas, who was even then engaged in suppressing yellow fever and controlling malaria in the Isthmus of Panama by destroying mosquitoes.)

Prevention had been extended into the human body itself. Immunization, an ancient folk remedy first used against smallpox, was bet-

6. Zinsser, *As I Remember Him*, 102.

ter understood and more widely applied, as doctors artificially stimu-
lated the body's immune system by injecting weakened or dead
microbes. Sometimes sera from the blood of animals that had been infected with a disease might be injected, carrying the antibodies formed
by the animal's immune system. Still rare in the medical arsenal were
"specifics"—chemicals that attacked a particular illness or reduced its
symptoms, as quinine did for malaria.

Improved diagnosis, aseptic surgery, and triumphs in preventive
medicine were the hallmarks of the time as Stan settled down to his
studies at Hopkins. The excitement of a new age lingered: "Light from
all the sciences," said the bacteriologist Hans Zinsser, "was bringing
never-suspected correlations; and a lovely orderliness was emerging
from the fog."[7]

Hopkins was a businesslike place. Lecturers were apt to assume, as
Welch did, that the students knew the book, and go on from there. To
Stan the laboratories looked "palatial," though they were so only in
comparison to Sheffield and Tulane. The rooms were high-ceilinged,
cold in winter; investigators blew their own glassware and did simple
repairs on their instruments. The students lacked the devil-may-care
attitude Stan had noticed at Tulane; they expected to discipline themselves and to be dealt with sharply if they did not.[8]

Like the other students, Stan encountered the varied sides of the
profession. Surgery he found "interesting . . . but not attractive." *Appalling* was a better word. His first exposure had come at Charity Hospital in New Orleans, when he was still at Tulane. Someone began to
cut the bandages from a woman patient preparatory to surgery, and
Stan "hit the floor in a dead faint right away." At Hopkins, surgery was
above all the province of William Halsted, who had introduced rubber

7. *Ibid.*, 111; Harry F. Dowling, *Fighting Infection* (Cambridge, Mass., 1977), especially 1–124. Useful histories of Bayne-Jones's future specialty include William Bullock, *A
History of Bacteriology* (1938; rpr., London, 1960); Hubert A. Lechevalier and Morris Solotorovsky, *Three Centuries of Microbiology* (New York, 1965); and W. D. Foster, *A History of
Medical Bacteriology and Immunology* (London, 1970).
8. Phillips interview, 70–73.

gloves into the operating room in the 1890s. The tall, balding surgeon, too formidable to be called a dandy, wore clothes crafted in Europe, and his house featured antiques and bowing servants. But Halsted's work was no less bloody than any other surgeon's. On the bleacher-like high stands where students sat to watch the cutting, Stan became nauseated and almost fell off. Enough was enough—he never felt tempted to pursue surgery.[9]

Medicine was another matter. Even as a student in the second year, he began to substitute for the clinical clerks on the hospital wards whenever he could, obeying Welch's dictum that "the care of the sick stands first, and is never to be forgotten, for the welfare of the patient is the primary purpose of the hospital." But Hopkins' roots also ran deep into the research-oriented German system, and Stan was soon absorbed in laboratory work as well. Carrying over German terminology, Hopkins encouraged each student to do an *arbeit,* seeking the solution to some problem that seemed especially interesting. Stan's first effort grew out of his summer's work in physiology at Chicago; after Howell excused him from repeating the course at Hopkins, he spent the time doing original work on the complex process by which blood coagulates.

In all, Stan put in a year of intermittent effort in "a little room of [Howell's] laboratory," working on the extraction of prothrombin—a substance from which the coagulating agent thrombin is derived—from platelets. Howell outlined the problem and guided every step of the effort. Stan reviewed the literature, did the work, and wrote up his results. He listed his professor as principal author, but after revising the essay to make it publishable, Howell quietly lined out his own name. When the result appeared in the *American Journal of Physiology,* Stan, twenty-three years old and in his third year of medical school, was able to read his first contribution in print. Howell had given his student's career a helping hand, and Stan himself an object lesson in professional generosity.[10]

9. *Ibid.,* 88–89.
10. Flexner and Flexner, *William Henry Welch,* 59; Stanhope Bayne-Jones, "The Presence of Prothrombin and Thromboplastin in the Blood Platelets," *American Journal of Physiology,* XXX (1912), 74–79. As clinical clerks, third- and fourth-year students were as-

His second publication, this time emerging from the clinical laboratory at Hopkins, was a simplified way to enable the general practitioner to test urine for chlorides. Stan's report on this practical bit of analytical chemistry, relating Hopkins' labs to general practice, came complete with multiple tables and overweighty explanation, which, quite as much as its modest and useful topic, may have helped to win it publication. Before he had his M.D., Stan had caught the eye of medical editors. "I am writing to those men," said one, pleading for submissions, "whose work I know will make good copy." When Stan was an intern, another editor wrote to praise his "excellent English" and ability to present a paper in "admirable form." Throughout his career, Stan was to do both important and unimportant papers, but he seldom failed to achieve publication in either case. A large and constantly expanding bibliography helped to establish his professional credentials in the burgeoning age of scientific medicine.[11]

But his profession meant also a wide acquaintance with the human staples of misery and need. The hospital's only community health service was in obstetrics. As a fourth-year student, Stan went out to deliver children in the poorer quarters of Baltimore, under the supervision of an instructor. Thus he encountered an ugly city where life was harsh. On one such outing, a poor Jewish woman named Salzberg, who earned her bread by ironing in a Chinese laundry, gave birth before Stan's instructor showed up. Stan delivered the child—his first delivery, though fortunately not her first—and was cleaning up afterward, when to his amazement a second child emerged. He went back to work, "tied the cord and cut it off and cleaned things."

Afterward he returned on postpartum visits, carrying his little black bag. The twins developed unevenly, one robust and the other "a wizened little thing." The woman wanted to name one after him, and he chose the weak one, assuming it would die and end the connection. Instead, the strong one died, and Stanhope Bayne Salzberg lived on. Until after World War I, when he lost track of the family, he clothed

---

signed a few beds; they took histories, performed such basic procedures as changing dressings, and did physical examinations. See Ludmerer, *Learning to Heal*, 60.

11. Stanhope Bayne-Jones, "Simplified Methods for Quantitative Estimation of Chlorids [*sic*] in the Urine," *Archives of Internal Medicine*, XII (1913), 90–111; Eustis to Bayne-Jones, January 8, 1914, and Janeway to Bayne-Jones, July 20, 1915, in A-34, Box 8, SBJC.

and fed his namesake and contributed as well to the care of an older sister and two brothers, one of whom was crippled.[12]

Stan received his M.D. in the spring of 1914, standing first in his class and winning a warm note of praise from Welch. He remained at Hopkins as an intern in the hospital, learning some of his own limitations, as well as the quirks of the doctors who did ward rounds. He kept to the medical wards, swapping them about with the other interns. The long hours devoured his time. "This is actual work now," he wrote his sister Marian, "to which the work I have done when I substituted here before seems now mere child's play. There is lots today—and not much sleep."

Both patients and doctors taught him much. Ward F was full of West Virginia miners; Stan recognized their suffering, their isolation in the city, and tried to talk to them. But his pale fine hair and unlined face did not encourage confidence, and the miners growled, "We came down here to see a doctor, not a child!" Among the doctors who used this human material for teaching purposes, Stan observed both compassion and coldness, honesty and showmanship. One physician, leading his students through the ward, would take the patients at random and struggle toward a diagnosis; another would preselect a case, read up on the illness in advance, and dazzle his admirers with his knowledge. Meanwhile, the intern, who knew how the trick was done, stood by and held his peace.

Stan continued to work in the labs. He participated in a study in which an associate, L. G. Rowntree, used an opaque substance, iodoform oil, to enable X rays to be made of the lungs—some genuine pioneering there, though Stan always gave Rowntree the credit for it. At the hospital, a case of a patient whose viscera were displaced into the chest cavity not only won Stan another publication but brought him into contact with Max Broedel, a German medical illustrator who had been invited to America by one of the Hopkins staff. Broedel's elegant drawings embellished several of Stan's publications, adding grace as well as clarity to his work.[13]

12. Phillips interview, 100–101; Bayne-Jones to Edith Denegre, October 5, 1917, in B-2, Box 8, SBJC.

13. Bayne-Jones to Marian, September 6, 1914, in A-34, Box 8, SBJC; A. A. Waters, S. Bayne-Jones, and L. G. Rowntree, "Roentgenography of the Lungs. Roentgenographic

Stan's social life also took on a medical cast. Broedel was well attuned not only to Hopkins but to Baltimore's large German community. A brewer by trade, a musician as well as an artist, he was a friend of H. L. Mencken's and the proprietor of an agreeable *bierstube*. Here, on Saturday nights, Stan and his friends from the hospital gathered to imbibe and sing, while Broedel and Mencken played doubles on the piano.[14]

Other aspects of Stan's work led him back to his forebears. Welch, a scholar as well as a scientist, preached the value of medical history and helped to reawaken his fascination with Joseph Jones. In 1890 William Osler had founded the Johns Hopkins University Historical Club; Welch became its first president, and during 1913 the club met on Saturday nights at the Surgeon-General's Library in Washington. Stan delivered papers at meetings and by 1914 had decided to write his grandfather's life. Here was the beginning of a lifelong hobby, rooted in personal memory and family pride rather than the strict concerns of objective scholarship.[15]

Hard-worked and maturing rapidly, Stan became, like many a doctor, engrossed in medicine almost to the exclusion of other things. In this absorbing profession, writes a social scientist, the physician finds "all the mental stimulation, the call upon his imagination, the contact with human life and human suffering, which his personality requires . . . and unending outlets for his inner capacities." Stan thought that he knew where his work was taking him—back to New Orleans; to a practitioner's life like his grandfather's; to hard but agreeable work; to an impecunious but respectable existence.

"I would be answering a tinkle bell like he did," he thought, admitting patients into an office in a room of his home. Or was that really why he had come to Hopkins?[16]

Studies in Living Animals after Intratracheal Injection of Iodoform Emulsion," *Archives of Internal Medicine*, XIX (1917), 538–49; Bayne-Jones, "Eventration of the Diaphragm," *Archives of Internal Medicine*, XVII (1916), 221–37.

14. Phillips interview, 76–77.

15. *Ibid.*, 68. On the biography of Joseph Jones, see also materials in Box 1, Folder 1, SBJT.

16. Garceau, *Political Life of the AMA*, 62; Phillips interview, 78.

He stood, after all, close to the heart of the growing tradition of scientific medicine. He had already won notice for his own research, and he had Welch for a patron. Stan's thoughts of becoming a general practitioner began to slip away in the summer of 1915 when Johns Hopkins, with the aim of retaining him despite a residency offered by Bellevue, selected him for a Rockefeller-financed post as assistant resident pathologist. At the same time, Stan was accepted as a candidate for the degree of master of arts in pathology.

His new position kept him in the Hopkins community and in Baltimore, where by now he had many ties. His post brought him into a field that had pioneered basic advances in medical research, and it brought him closer, not so much to the life that Joseph Jones had actually led, as to the one he would have liked to lead, had he not been born in the wrong country and sixty years too soon. Yet hidden within Welch's apparent gift and the lure of the laboratory was the danger that the path Stan was following might not be his own, but the ideal of his two ideals.[17]

By 1916 he was already moving away from medical practice and from his father's life. Events at Hopkins now drove him further. The resident pathologist was Baltimore-born Milton C. Winternitz. He was a Welch student, "a steam engine in pants," a tiny man physically but brilliant, brusque, and domineering. In 1915 his remarkable energies focused on a project for a New Hunterian Laboratory.

The original Hunterian—the name derived from the great eighteenth century English surgeon, John Hunter—was a small structure on the medical school grounds. Established in 1905, the laboratory was divided between the departments of surgery and pathology. In the surgical section, third-year students spent their Fridays practicing on animals under realistic operating-room conditions. The animals were, of course, anesthetized, and careful records were kept, as with human patients; if the dog or cat died, a full postmortem was done on the remains. The Old Hunterian also provided services in veterinary surgery to Baltimore pet owners, from whom the doctors, ever alert to attacks by antivivisectionists, were careful to collect testimonials. (The

17. On appointments, see materials in A-34, Box 8, SBJC.

neurosurgeon Harvey Cushing, moving spirit behind the original laboratory, later recalled winning over the most militant of local antivivisectionists by removing a tumor from her pet poodle.)

By 1916 a committee on the new laboratory was formed with Winternitz as chairman, and by the end of the year funds from the General Education Board of the John D. Rockefeller Fund enabled a building to rise on the northwest corner of the medical school lot, with additional facilities for medicine, surgery, and pediatrics.[18] Winternitz wanted to establish a division of his pathology lab—for which the creation of the New Hunterian had made room—to deal with bacteriology and immunology. He launched a vigorous fund-raising campaign that brought in the requisite $22,500 to fund the effort for three years, exploiting private philanthropists, drug houses, and insurance companies as sources of cash. Winternitz then began a lengthy and fruitless search for a top name in the field, to head the division.

In plain fact, Hopkins wanted a lot and had little to offer in return. Despite Winternitz' talk of basic discoveries to come from the new division, his primary aim was to serve the hospital. Lack of a laboratory resulted in bacteriological studies being farmed out in makeshift fashion to other departments. Winternitz wanted from his top man not only research but teaching and much routine work for the hospital as well—and he could guarantee funding for only three years. Not surprisingly, well-established men had better positions already, and one by one all turned him down. Thus Winternitz turned at last to his resident, announcing in March 1916 that Dr. Stanhope Bayne-Jones (A.B. Yale, 1910, M.D. Johns Hopkins, 1914) had been appointed director.

There was, of course, a problem pointed out by Stan's later remark, "Well, I had never had anything but an ordinary course in bacteriology up to that time." To his contributors, Winternitz announced that Stan was "well equipped to carry on the work." In fact he was not

18. Arthur J. Viseltear, "Milton C. Winternitz and the Yale Institute of Human Relations: A Brief Chapter in the History of Social Medicine," *Yale Journal of Biology and Medicine*, LVII (1984), 869. On Winternitz, see also Chapter Six, below, and Dan A. Oren, *Joining the Club: A History of Jews at Yale* (New Haven, 1985), 139–43. On laboratories, see materials in file on Hunterian Laboratory Correspondence, Animal Receipts, December, 1916–April, 1917; Harvey Cushing to Jay McLean, January 24, 1920, in file on Hunterian Laboratory—Old; photocopy of letter, Wallace Buttrick to R. Brent Keyser, July 3, 1914, in file on New Hunterian Laboratory, all in AMC.

well equipped at all. To make him ready, Hopkins sent him posthaste to six months of study at Columbia University's College of Physicians and Surgeons under one of the nation's new stars, Hans Zinsser—"the best man in this field engaged in teaching in this country," said Welch. By the end of the month, Stan was occupying another of his transient abodes, this time in Manhattan.[19]

Zinsser was one of the memorable figures of the German-American scientific culture that helped to transplant European medical science to American soil. He was the son of German immigrants and about a decade older than Stan. Handsome and charming, a hard driver at work, given to volcanic rages, Zinsser was also a brave, humorous, and many-talented man. Not without magnetism himself, Stan recognized a more matured and brilliant form of the same power at work in the medical school on 59th Street, and paid it homage. "I went to Dr. Zinsser's department and was charmed beyond resistance by . . . his vivid personality and energy, ideas and ranging mind." Baffled by a problem, Zinsser, like Sherlock Holmes, would seize his violin and fiddle things into perspective. He was writing a textbook of bacteriology that would remain a standard for generations.[20]

In short order, Stan had become "Jonesie" to his new mentor. Under Zinsser, he plunged into a concentrated study of the microscopic world that had beguiled his father. Despite all superficial differences, the immigrant's child and the low-keyed, ingratiating southerner agreed in basics, including their appetites for science and life. In March, 1916, after Stan had returned to Hopkins, Zinsser wrote him: "Dear Jonsie [sic]:—Would you, under any circumstances, consider coming here as Assistant Professor with me?" He offered only $2,000 a year and acknowledged that Stan's "splendid opportunities" at Hopkins made him recognize that his offer was a "long shot."[21]

In fact, Johns Hopkins was not to have Stan for long. And yet his

19. William H. Welch to Bayne-Jones, March 8, 1916, in A-34, Box 8, SBJC; see also Milton C. Winternitz to Jencks, Van Wort, White et al., June 18, [1915], and to his contributors, March, 1916. Winternitz' real views on the services the Bacteriology and Immunology Division was to provide are reflected in his letter to Winford H. Smith, Superintendent, The Johns Hopkins Hospital, March 6, 1915. All in A-35, Box 8, SBJC. See also Phillips interview, 79.

20. Phillips interview, 79.

21. Hans Zinsser to Bayne-Jones, March 29, 1916, in A-34, Box 8, SBJC.

last year there before the war was a busy and happy one. Heading up the new division of Winternitz' laboratory, he began to instruct medical students in bacteriology, replacing an older man who had failed to reach them. Stan succeeded by grasping the basic fact that his students were interested in disease. Where his predecessor had used harmless bacteria to demonstrate principles, Stan used bad actors—anthrax to show the formation of bacterial spores; the pneumococcus to demonstrate the importance of an organism's tough outer layer, or capsule. The result was "a burst of interest" on the part of the young people, for they were no longer learning abstractions; they were viewing the enemy and how he lived and defended himself. Stan had taken his first step toward mastering the teaching art.[22]

After five years in Baltimore, Stan was a solid if very junior member of his profession. To stand first in his class, to be accepted as protégé by Welch and Zinsser in turn, to earn his master's degree in pathology and head the bacteriology section at Hopkins—all marked a career begun on the fast track. At the same time, he abandoned seemingly without a sigh the life of the practitioner that absorbed most American doctors. He was an academic full-timer, a physician whose world was the laboratory and the lecture room. Joseph Jones had longed for a life in research without being able to pursue it. Now Stan had attained it at the beginning of his career. But already circumstances were calling him to practice a completely different kind of medicine, far from the comfortable city on the Chesapeake.

The instinct for soldiering is said to go deep in southern men. Members of Stan's family—including both grandfathers—had worn the gray. His uncle Hamilton Jones had gone to the Spanish-American War as a battalion surgeon. His own interest in the military may have begun with family war stories and with the arms and armor in Joseph Jones's collection. He remembered, too, a hot day in 1898 when, from the Denegres' yard, he watched columns of men march by on their way to the docks, to take ship for Cuba.[23]

22. Phillips interview, 86.
23. *Ibid.*, 120.

But for all this martial tradition, Stan came of age in a peaceful world. His first view of Europe, as a nineteen-year-old tourist shepherded by Tante E, had featured cathedrals, French watering places, Rhine castles, and other guidebook wonders. Later, people would look back on the decade before the war as the final warm afternoon of the old world. Of course that was hindsight: to a nineteen-year-old seeing Europe for the first time in 1908, the world was beginning, not ending. War seemed even more remote when Stan returned to America, and he passed through his first quarter-century without donning a uniform.

His closest personal connection with the Army was through "Uncle Willy" Gorgas, whose mother had been Stan's great-aunt. As a child, William Crawford Gorgas had seen Robert E. Lee and Stonewall Jackson confer with his father in the front parlor of the family home in Richmond. Decades later, as a young army surgeon in Texas, he had contracted yellow fever, survived, and—because a bout of the disease conferred lifelong immunity—was thereafter likely to be sent by the surgeon general wherever Yellow Jack appeared; hence his posting to Cuba. Though he doubted Walter Reed's discovery that mosquitoes carried the disease, Gorgas systematically worked out the methods necessary to destroy the vector. To the astonishment of all, himself included, his work freed Havana of yellow fever for the first time in centuries.

Then he was assigned as chief sanitary officer to the Isthmus of Panama, where yellow fever and malaria threatened to defeat American efforts to build a transoceanic canal. Informed by the discoveries of the past generation, Gorgas embodied in scientific form a tradition of military preventive medicine whose remote origins can be traced to biblical times. By imposing the latest knowledge with military discipline he became a lifesaver of heroic proportions among the legion of engineers, soldiers, and Caribbean workers who built the canal.[24]

In response to an invitation from Gorgas, Stan spent some lively months in Panama during the summer of 1912. His visit (according to his later account) began with a stroke of luck. While waiting on the dock

24. Marie D. Gorgas and Burton J. Hendrick, *William Crawford Gorgas: His Life and Work* (New York, 1924); William C. Gorgas, *Sanitation in Panama* (New York, 1915); David McCullough, *The Path Between the Seas: The Creation of the Panama Canal, 1870–1914* (New York, 1977), 411.

at Colón for the customs inspectors to finish with his luggage, Stan spied a tattered pamphlet on the floor and picked it up. It was a reprint of an article on *Schistosoma mansoni*, an intestinal parasite. He read it idly, largely through a habit he had acquired at Hopkins of reading anything printed that came along. Then he boarded the little train that ran to Panama on the Pacific Coast and, arriving in the dark, found himself a bed in the bachelors' quarters where he spent a hot, restless night, turning and scratching.

Morning revealed a blood-streaked sheet, a population of bed-bugs, and a greasy pillow where other heads had lain. He hastened to his assigned post in a big ward of the hospital that held black laborers, about ninety sick men. There the medical officer, who thought he knew what second-year students were good for, set him to examining 250 specimens of feces in a small room on the second floor, under a tin roof. The place stank like a dunghill and had the temperature of an oven.

Stan began smearing feces on slides and contemplating the result through a microscope. The third or fourth contained a "perfectly beautiful" spined egg that Stan recognized at once. He had seen it the day before in an illustration in the pamphlet on *Schistosoma mansoni*. He wrote his finding down in the diagnostic book, assuming that if he could identify the egg, anyone could. The doctors could not. Finding his note in the book during ward rounds, several hastened to Stan's oven to view the specimen. Then they called in Samuel T. Darling, the chief pathologist of the Canal Zone, who confirmed the diagnosis. "And so the attitude . . . turned from one of contempt to respect, and I was given a white coat and a stethoscope and allowed to come down and be a doctor."

On his days off, he accompanied Gorgas to see mosquito control work and the canal. One day Gorgas and Stan, accompanied by a second youth, started out for Miraflores. They walked along a railroad embankment because the muddy waters of Gatun Lake were rising about them. Iguanas roosted in the branches of trees, and big tarantulas clung to sticks rising from the flood. Soon the lake covered the embankment, and the men, holding their watches and cameras overhead, continued to wade until the water rose chest high.

Suddenly the embankment disappeared beneath them. A railroad bridge over a little valley had been removed, and they were struggling in forty feet of turbulent water. Stan clung to his watch and camera until Gorgas shouted, "You fool, let them go!"

They thrashed about among the thin top branches of the trees. The embankment was somewhere, but where? For a time they roosted in separate trees that stood above the flood. Then Gorgas plunged back in and found the embankment. He called the others, and they swam to join him. Soaked and exhausted, they had a hard walk home, for they had kicked off their shoes and the embankment was thick with brambles.[25]

Reflecting on his adventure, Stan found that he liked the taste of danger. The curiosity and fearlessness that had led him into the attics of the house on Howard Avenue had not changed. The excess energy that had gone into tantrums and misbehavior as a child was still with him as a man. The discovery was important, for two summers later the world quite suddenly became a more dangerous place.

In August, 1914, he was home on vacation, sitting on the porch at Biloxi, when he heard the news that war had broken out in Europe. The Denegres were deeply affected: France was a sentimental homeland; Napoleon was almost a living presence in their house, "the greatest law giver and the greatest military leader in the world." During the months that followed, early hopes for a short war faded into the reality of a protracted, bloody stalemate on the Western Front. In June, 1915, Stan received a letter from Gorgas, now surgeon general of the Army. "I would like to have you in the Army Medical Reserve Corps. . . . Have you ever considered the question of making an application?"

In the volunteer army of those times, the medical reserve officer could be called to duty only with his own consent, receiving in that case $166.66 a month, or $2,000 a year. In mid-July, Stan applied for his appointment; a week later he appeared for examination, was found qualified, and commissioned on August 7, 1915.[26]

Soon the itch for action set in. The spring of 1916 found American

25. Phillips interview, 80–84.
26. William Crawford Gorgas to Bayne-Jones, June 17 and June 29, 1915, in B-1, Box 8, SBJC; U.S. Army Medical Department, *Circular of Information*, May 23, 1908, *ibid.* See also DA Form 66, Item 12, in Bayne-Jones's 201 File, Federal Personnel Records Center, St. Louis. Some official records erroneously give his date of rank one year early.

troops operating along the Mexican border in response to raids by Pancho Villa. Apparently Stan asked for an assignment; the call came while he was living in New York and working with Zinsser. A regiment of the Maryland National Guard, called to federal duty, had pitched its tents in a field near the racetrack in Laurel. Stan joined the unit for a few weeks and then fell ill, apparently with infectious hepatitis. He returned to his room in New York and tried to work but could not. Weak and jaundiced, he was admitted to Presbyterian Hospital until he recovered. His first brush with field service had ended, like many another young soldier's, with a camp disease.[27]

But in April, 1917, after years of increasing acrimony, the United States severed diplomatic relations with the German Empire over the issue of unrestricted submarine warfare. Shortly afterward, Congress declared war. Stan, now a newly promoted reserve captain, was at work in his fifth-floor laboratory at Hopkins when he heard the news. Soon Welch invited him to spend the war in Baltimore, training bacteriologists for the Army. Stan agreed.

Yet the decision left him unsatisfied. He was twenty-eight years old, and he had been going to school, either as student or teacher, for most of his life. He had a spirit, an eye for adventure, a degree of physical courage appropriate to a more active life than the one he had led thus far. He traveled down to Washington, to the old multicolumned State, War, and Navy Building on Pennsylvania Avenue next to the White House, where Gorgas had his office. Ostensibly, he had come to ask Gorgas for the assignment Welch had recommended. "What was in my heart," Stan said later, "I really don't know."

But Gorgas spoke first. "Oh, Stan," he said, "I'm so glad to see you. Lord Balfour was in here a few minutes ago, and he said that they're desperately short of doctors for the British troops and battalions. I know you've got a uniform, and if you can get it out and get packed, I'll get you on a boat in five days."[28]

So at least Stan remembered the interview, many years later. He said nothing to Gorgas about the laboratory or the job proposed by

27. William Crawford Gorgas to Bayne-Jones, July, 1916, in A-34, Box 8, SBJC; Phillips interview, 116–17.
28. Phillips interview, 121.

Welch. Instead, he returned to Baltimore and told Welch that he was going to war. Whatever his own views, Welch had not become one of the country's greatest teachers without knowing when to let a young man go his way. That way now led to one of the great battlefields of 1917, to Passchendaele and the wet Flanders plain.

FOUR

The Making of a Soldier

From the early months of the war in 1914, American doctors and nurses went to Europe as volunteers to aid England and France. When Congress declared war, doctors and nurses were again among the first to go. Great Britain wanted medical assistance, and units maintained by American hospitals and medical schools answered the call.[1]

A few individual reservists went too, Stan among them. Joining Base Hospital No. 4 from Cleveland's Lakeside Hospital on board the Cunard liner SS *Orduna,* he sailed on May 8, 1917, full of exhilaration over his coming part in the "great human experience of the war." The weather was in tune; except for two rough days, the sky was fresh and bright, full of the North Atlantic spring, when the air seems to glitter with salt.[2]

The Americans' arrival was triumphant. King George V and Queen Mary received them in the garden of Buckingham Palace, amid a Gainsborough-like setting of green lawns and noble trees. Then the officers enjoyed tea at the American embassy. On the streets, "everyone you meet is a friend," wrote Stan, as the English flocked to greet these men and women whom they rightly saw as down payment on greater American forces to come.[3]

In short order the unit moved on to France. Stan, pining for action, went to the medical director of his region and declared that he wanted to serve with the troops, not with the hospital. The next day, warning orders came. He went through brief schooling to learn the use

1. On the early efforts, see Harvey Cushing, *From a Surgeon's Journal, 1915–1918* (Boston, 1936), 3–55; W. A. R. Chapin, *The Lost Legion* (Springfield, Mass., 1926); and Grace Crile, ed., *George Crile, An Autobiography* (Philadelphia, 1947), I, 247–55.

2. Telegram, Bayne-Jones to Mrs. George Denegre, May 8, 1917, and letter, Bayne-Jones to Mrs. George Denegre, May 17, 1917, in GDC. On the American base hospitals, see P. M. Ashburn, *A History of the Medical Department of the United States Army* (Boston, 1929), 322.

3. New York *Times,* May 24 [25?], 1917; London *Times,* May 24, 1917; Bayne-Jones to Tante E, May 23, 1917, in B-2, Box 8, SBJC.

of the gas mask—in those times a clumsy rubber contraption that covered the whole face, with a clip for the nose like a clothespin, and a respirator the size of a knapsack that hung against the chest. When his final orders came on June 19, the Clevelanders gave him a fine send-off, with soup, champagne, and speeches. Next morning he packed his haversack and rolled up the rest of his belongings in his blanket, off at last for his "paradoxical El Dorado," the front.

For twenty-four hours he bumped along in a train, arriving in Belgium at a blank "muddy little place" somewhere close to the much-battered town of Ypres. He slept in a tent, to be waked at two the next morning by a sergeant looming behind a lighted lantern. A Ford flivver converted into an ambulance waited outside. Squeaking merrily, it delivered him to his new outfit, the 69th Field Ambulance, 23rd Division, British Expeditionary Forces.[4]

For the moment, the unit was in reserve. Billeted in a farmhouse, Stan could hear the guns, still far enough away to be merely interesting. The field ambulance was the basic unit of medical care in the British army; three such units, with two companies of stretcher-bearers and orderlies each, supported every division. At the 69th Stan learned his first lessons in how to survive, and help others to survive, in combat.

Then he moved up to the line. He had his first taste of being shelled at an advanced dressing station in the open, and then in a dug-out that trembled under the impact of the explosions. He learned to recognize the "queer, whistling, wobbly sound" of a gas shell, the small bang at the end of its trip. "I have not been as scared as I thought I would be," he noted, even though "the war is horrible beyond imagination."

It was so especially for the wounded. Casualties traveled from the front by litter to a rear assembly point, by division stretcher bearers to a central station, by "trolley" to the divisional collection post, and by motor ambulance to the advanced dressing station. Poison gas tormented them and those who cared for them. Stan worked for long hours in his mask, "sweating, half suffocated, dribbling, hardly able to see through the eye pieces that get so steaming." Under a barrage, he and an En-

4. Bayne-Jones to Tante E, June 23, 1917, in B-2, Box 8, SBJC; Phillips interview, 128–29. See also Archibald Frank Becke, comp., *Order of Battle of Divisions: Part I, The Regular British Divisions* (London, 1935), 119–25.

glish captain huddled together, like millions of soldiers for three years past, in a stinking verminous hole. Then, returning to the open, they resumed their duties among "dead horses, dead men, feces everywhere."

In his first tour on the line, Stan was under fire for twenty days. On July 23, his unit marched, singing, twelve miles back through the hot dust to a little village near the border of France and Belgium, where they rested. Stan marched with them, wearing the same clothes he had set out in—itching, lousy, and a veteran.[5]

Now, as a regimental surgeon with a battalion of the 11th Sherwood Foresters to supervise, his work emphasized the inglorious duties of preventive medicine. Stan supervised sanitation, examined men for venereal disease, and held morning sick parade ("A dose of castor oil . . . sometimes works wonders in cooling a man's ardour for Sick parade," counseled his manual). He had to keep a Regimental Aid Post Diary of diagnoses, treatment, and disposal of patients; a Sanitary Diary of his recommendations for unit sanitation and actions taken to correct defects; a roll of cooks and men employed in handling food stores; a roll of officers and men with enteric complaints; and a record of inoculations.

All this was a long way from the excitement of war he had looked forward to, but—as he was to say many years later—wars are won by the healthy, and under such conditions the conventional medical preoccupation with curing misses the point. On the Western Front preventive medicine was especially critical. For centuries surgeons had known that no form of warfare was more likely to produce epidemics than a siege, when two armies, immobilized, lived crowded together among their own wastes. Here the war had precisely the character of an immense and interminable siege, and without rigorous medical discipline the troops could hardly have escaped devastating outbreaks of disease.

Besides his duties in keeping his men healthy, Stan prepared to aid them when they were sick or wounded. Again army paper work was heavy: He had to make out sick reports, tallies of the wounded, "indents," or requisitions for stores, medical records on which men were to be evacuated and why, and notes on self-inflicted wounds for court-martial testimony.

5. Bayne-Jones to Uncle George, July 24, 1917, in B-2, Box 8, SBJC; Phillips interview, 130; 23rd Division Medical Arrangements No. 112, . . . 11th September 1917, in B-6, Box 8, SBJC.

During battle, Stan learned that he must establish an Advanced Aid Post where the wounded could be gathered, while remaining himself at the Regimental Aid Post (the battalion aid station, in American terminology), the first spot where casualties saw a doctor. He must do everything possible to ensure that the injured were found and brought in, must give them first aid and send them on to the main dressing station of the field ambulance. To accomplish his varied duties, he commanded two orderlies; his batman, or personal servant; an NCO and eight men to perform sanitary duties; an NCO and four men to perform "water duty"; and an NCO and sixteen men as stretcher-bearers.[6]

Gradually mastering his duties, he found that he had what he wanted, "a great job—and rather lively." He had in the soldiers of the line almost the only patients he would ever serve directly. As he said, his duty was "to take care of the men where they are in the most trouble." He felt at peace, even though his work, a routine of observation and patchwork, meant nothing as Johns Hopkins understood medicine: merely "cleaning out pieces and things, putting bandages on and stopping bleeding."

But Stan had "lost interest in [scientific] medicine and bugs—temporarily." In place of the laboratory and the classroom he had the touch of humanity and the taste of danger, and he was unsure which he valued most. "The action and excitement," he said, "and [the] wild chances are what make all this worth while to me."[7]

After a spell of rain and mud the weather broke and summer returned to the Belgian border. The days were almost tender, with shrapnel bursts drifting like bits of down across the deep blue sky. Stan was far from everything he had ever known, and at times when he was not busy, home and his family filled his thoughts and assumed a new perspective. He felt closer than ever to his sister Marian, and admitted her into his thoughts more deeply than anyone else.

6. Capt. T. R. H. Blake, "The Duties of a Regimental Medical Officer," in B-6, Box 8, SBJC. See also "Medical Organization in the Field" and "Clerical Work of a Regimental Medical Officer," n.d., *ibid*. A British regiment was an organizational and recruiting device rather than a tactical unit.

7. Bayne-Jones to George Denegre, August 26, and Bayne-Jones to Marian, August 12, 1917, in B-2, Box 8, SBJC; Phillips interview, 132–33.

One blazing day he tipped a borrowed chair against the wall of a farmhouse to write her a letter. He blinked at the sun glaring on the paper and suddenly, with a stab of homesickness, recollected the sun on the sand and the shell roads at Biloxi. He dreamed of the contentment, if he survived, of settling down as a professor somewhere, probably at Hopkins, with a house of his own and "some one I may find brave enough to risk my bad disposition." He hoped that after the war he would not be so inhuman as in the past: "that notion about the sand at Biloxi has made me sentimental."[8]

For home news, he depended most upon Edith. Tante E, putting aside invalidism for the duration of the war, had plunged enthusiastically into Belgian relief—for which she was later decorated by the Belgian government—and into war work with the Travellers' Aid. She sought Gorgas' help to stamp out prostitution in Biloxi (no easy task then or later). She made sure that the center of the family held, copying and passing letters on to keep its far-flung members aware of each other's doings. Needing these contacts as never before, Stan often sounded a note of reconciliation in his own letters. "What I've been through," he wrote his foster parents, "has made me more than ever tender of the good things you . . . have done for me."[9]

Then his unit returned to the line. The great battle of Passchendaele had begun, and the 11th Sherwood Foresters joined the British push somewhere near the Ypres-Menin road, where German pillboxes made the advance slow and costly. The weather turned foul, and the coldest and wettest summer on record set in; the ground became muck, the wounded sometimes drowned where they fell, and litterbearers struggled with their burdens over duckboards.

When shells began to fall, Stan lay in the mud while the ground leaped like the surface of a pond under rain. The mud was also thick inside the captured German bunker where he received the wounded;

8. Bayne-Jones to Marian, August 12, 1917, in B-2, Box 8, SBJC.

9. Bayne-Jones to George Denegre, August 26, 1917, Hugh Bayne to George Denegre, September 2, 1917, Edith's note accompanying a transcription of Bayne-Jones to George Denegre, September 10, 1917, all in B-2, Box 8, SBJC. Materials on Edith's doings in Box 6, Gorgas Papers, Library of Congress.

the flies on the walls swarmed over one another, while all about and overhead the earth was "beaten by huge steel flails" as the bombardment moved ahead of a German counterattack.[10]

This was war at its most brutal and medicine at its most basic. One day an Australian, holding one forearm with the other hand, came into the bloody culvert that was Stan's aid station. While Stan cut with a scissors the last threads of flesh that bound the arm on, the soldier said, "I stopped a five point nine with my elbow." Responsibility burdened Stan's spirit. At four every morning, when the firing quieted enough to let the stretcher-bearers out, he triaged the wounded. As many as twelve men were needed to manage a single litter over the mucky, cratered ground. Not all the wounded could be moved, and the hard rule of triage was to save those who might survive and let the others die. At that unearthly hour, in the stinking tunnel, Stan had to play God and decide who went and who did not.

When autumn came the great battle wound down at last. The British had paid 238,313 casualties for control of a ridgeline that did not prove to be particularly valuable. Then the Germans, victorious over Russia, shifted troops southward to aid their Austrian allies, inflicting a crushing defeat on the Italians at Caporetto. French and British troops rushed to the front, and Stan went with them.

Packed into fifty-nine trains, the 23rd Division rolled for five days on a thousand-mile journey. Men resurrected from the Flanders mud gazed unbelievingly at "terraced vineyards and glorious, tree-clad slopes, in all the bravery of their autumn tints," as they crossed the Midi. Stan's element detrained at Mantua and, with every button polished, marched to the line.[11]

10. Bayne-Jones to Tante E, October 3 and October 17, 1917, in B-2, Box 8, SBJC. On the general history of the battle, see Brig. Gen. Sir James E. Edmonds, ed., *Military Operations in France and Belgium—1917* (London, 1948), 279, Vol. II of *History of the Great War*, 6 vols. This is part of the official history, which attempts to portray Passchendaele as a success for the British, albeit a modest one. The 23rd Division suffered a total of 2,134 casualties during September 20–25, 1917.

11. Robert J. Blackham, *Scalpel, Sword and Stretcher: Forty Years of Work and Play* (London, n.d.), 270. Blackham was director of medical services for the 23rd Division—what Americans called a division surgeon.

In the hills north of Venice where the Piave runs through many channels out of the cold Dolomites, Allies and Austrians faced off on a front settling into immobility as the Alpine winter shut down. Stan found the war "very slow out here." It was like Valley Forge, except that the men had boots and food. Snow powdered the hillsides, and the British huddled in deserted farmhouses or bivouacked in tents. Italian soldiers came out of the line, ragged and starving, and picked the fields bare. When they slept in a farmhouse, they defecated into their hands before leaving and flung the feces against the ceiling.

The Austrians were one to two thousand yards away (fifty to a hundred yards had been commoner in Flanders). No Man's Land was the Piave, an arroyo of boulders in the wintertime, when its water was locked up as snow on the Alpine heights. From beyond the river, the enemy occasionally lobbed big shells from thirteen-inch mortars, scattering the stones but doing little damage. The real foe was the weather; magnificent mountains loomed all around but were generally obscured by mist or erased by blowing snow; freezing and thawing made all footing slippery for men and beasts.

Monotony reigned as the cold did. When shells bean falling near the farmhouse where he kept his aid station, Stan and his stretcher-bearers went to work, scratching out a hole to hide in. (Very warming work, he found it, a help in saving his scanty firewood.) The main damage of the cannon was to the eardrums, for the roar echoed about the reverberating hills like thunder in the clouds. Stan thought of the way the sails of a schooner boomed, when a squall was coming up over the Gulf of Mexico, in the years when he had sailed with Bayne on green warm water.[12]

In this tedious desolation of snowy rock and cloud he needed more than ever his connections with home. He tried to explain to Marian why frontline soldiers rarely spoke of home to one another. "It is natural, of course, for us to repress emotions and to say little [i]f anything of what we think of our sister[s] and brothers and our families—and all the gentler desires for the natural peaceful life among our friends that this war has cut us off from. I've often seen that only when a man is hit

---

12. Bayne-Jones to Marian, January 2, 1918, in B-2, Box 8, SBJC. See also Bayne-Jones to Alma [Bayne's wife], January 17, 1918, and Bayne-Jones to Tante E, January 15, 1918, both *ibid*. See also Phillips interview, 140–41.

badly—got a wound that he probably won't recover from—does he talk about his people."[13]

Some Christmas boxes wended through to him. He filled up with pecans and good figs, searched for bread to sop up cane syrup, warmed himself in a pullover, and greased his face with Vaseline against the wind. Books sent by Tante E provided relief from having to read labels on jam and bully-beef tins. Further relief was provided by a leave in Rome. In March, 1918, Stan stayed with two English officers, friends from the Sherwood Foresters, at the Grand Hotel on the Piazza della Terme. The early Roman spring had already broken out in flowers; Americans thronged the city, and the Italians were cordial to their new allies. Stan and his friends attended parties, dinners, and the opera, played tennis nearly every day, and almost managed to forget the war.

But no sooner did he return to the Piave than long-expected orders came. The American Expeditionary Forces were now in France; as an American surgeon he was ordered to join them. He got the message in bivouac, weary and sweating after a two days' march, at the end of a dirt road. He packed up, got somehow to the nearest railhead, and boarded a train to Paris.

He went sorrowfully, leaving the officers and men with whom he had "shared a good many rough experiences," and his battalion, the only home he knew in the wasteland. He recognized that personal feelings counted for nothing: "[The war] makes you feel infinitesimal—but with all your feelings crammed intensely into that small bit of yourself that survives."[14]

In Paris he cleaned up at the Hotel Meurice on the Rue de Rivoli. Old friends were about; he spent some pleasant days with Uncle Hugh Bayne, encountered colleagues from Hopkins when he was posted to the AEF's Central Medical Department Laboratory at Dijon, and met Hans Zinsser, his teacher of bacteriology, now a colonel in the medical corps.

But Stan was as certain as ever of what he wanted to do. By now

13. Bayne-Jones to Marian, January 2, 1918, in B-2, Box 8, SBJC.
14. Bayne-Jones to Tante E, March 19, 1918, *ibid.* See also Bayne-Jones to Tante E, March 8, 1918, to "Nenaine," January 28, 1918, and to Tante E, February 14, 1918, all *ibid.*

he could have had no illusions about life on the line—the hard duty, the danger, and the lack of purely medical interest. Yet he began to agitate once again for a frontline post as a battalion surgeon. Paul de Kruif was also at Dijon, and years later he recalled a long walk he took with Stan—"this sandy-haired, open-faced, English-looking young American"—one night in the country. Not so much talking to de Kruif as thinking out loud, Stan argued that his duty was at the front, that fighting was more important than researching. "And next morning this strange, extreme opposite of a slacker pulled wires, and got himself ordered to the Yankee Division where, through the war, he took a doughboy's chances."

On March 29, relieved from his assignment with the lab, Stan moved to the 26th Division just as an immense new German offensive began. An organization of National Guard volunteers, the New Englanders of the Yankee Division had been holding a quiet sector of the line north of Soissons. Then they moved to the Toul sector, where Stan became surgeon of the 3rd Battalion, 101st Infantry, shifting on May 1 to the 2nd Battalion.[15]

American field medical organization differed only in detail from that of the British. The battalion aid station served as a collecting point for the wounded, staffed in theory by a surgeon, an assistant surgeon, a sergeant, and eight privates of the Medical Department. The surgeon's role was to apply first aid to the genuine casualties and to spot the malingerers. "Pills are not important [to the surgeon]," declared the AEF's *Weekly Bulletin of Disease;* "commonsense and all the qualities of a man are."

From the aid station the wounded were carried by litter to the ambulance head, to start their trip to a field hospital. There they were sorted into three groups, the sick, the wounded, and the gassed. They were also divided into transportables and nontransportables, and the former, after medical attention, were sent farther back to an evacuation hospital. Nontransportables passed into shock units where they might

15. Paul de Kruif, "I Collect People," *Ladies' Home Journal* October, 1941, p. 130. See also Order No. 23, Central Medical Department Laboratory, AEF, France, March 29, 1918, and Special Order No. 90, 26th Division, AEF, April 2, 1918, both in B-18, Box 9, SBJC. See also Frank M. Hume, *History of the 103rd U.S. Infantry: 1917–1919, 26th Division, A.E.F* (N.p., 103rd U.S. Infantry, 1919), 32; Albert E. George and Edwin H. Cooper, *Pictorial History of the Twenty-Sixth Division, United States Army* (Boston, 1920), 2–3.

receive blood transfusions from hospital personnel. Then followed stabilizing surgery by special teams, the grandfathers of the future MASH surgeons. The medical array was more elaborate than that of the British, but for the man at the bottom—the battalion surgeon—there was, except for the presence of the assistant battalion surgeon, little practical difference in duties and dangers.[16]

The 101st held a "hard bit of the line," said Stan, "—I should say a *soft* bit because it is nearly all mud, soft as soup and more than knee deep." The Germans occupied the hill of Montsec, rising out of the Woevre plain, and "look[ed] right down the throats of the Americans in [their] horrid sodden trenches." Stan's aid station stood in a once-pleasant village, now a jagged pile of stones, mortar, and cracked houses. To the north the Germans were advancing, having broken the front open after years of stalemate. Green American troops took over less active parts of the line, as French veterans rushed to the Second Battle of the Marne.[17]

For a little while Stan was able to write his letters quietly in a damp, candle-lit dugout, where the rain leaked slowly through the roof, and a charcoal fire glowed at his elbow. But his words were uneasy, filled with concern for the men in the cold trenches, who stood so deep in water that, unable to sleep, they were forced to catnap on the sodden firesteps. And as the foe's advance continued, he worried about the course of the fighting. "But—my God!—the German *can't* win this war!"[18]

Shifting to the 2nd Battalion, he encountered the problems of a still-amateur army trying to learn trench warfare. Americans were applying to their field medical service immense resources and the skills of their partly reformed medical profession. The upgrading of the medical schools at home meant better technical training for many of the young physicians, who were the ones most likely to be serving the troops. But if the potential was good, to Stan's veteran eye the practice was still grossly deficient. The American forces seemed almost entirely ignorant

16. Jay Weir Grissinger, *Medical Field Service in France* (Washington, 1928), 66–76; *Weekly Bulletin of Disease*, No. 17 (October 14, 1918), 5–6, in Box 3309, RG 120, NARA.

17. Bayne-Jones to Tante E, April 5, 1918, and Bayne-Jones to Uncle George, April 14, 1918, both in B-3, Box 8, SBJC. See also Phillips interview, 151.

18. Bayne-Jones to Marian, April 28, 1918, in B-3, Box 8, SBJC.

of elementary sanitation. Their position did not help: thirteen miles due east of St. Mihiel, spread out in the valley before Beaumont and holding the village of Seicheprey, they occupied a sector where the 102nd Infantry had lately undergone a German attack.

Trenches and dugouts had been destroyed, and the shell-plowed, rubble-strewn earth was littered with decaying food, rusting tin cans, and human feces. One company of the 101st lived in a long tunnel driven into a hillside, which served also as a latrine and a dump for discarded equipment. Rubber boots were delivered late, and meanwhile the men in the trenches waded in leather shoes and canvas puttees through a stew of mud and excrement one to three feet deep—in short, an Augean stable, and getting a cleanup started was Stan's first duty.[19]

American soldiers also needed training against gas. After cleaning up the 2nd Battalion, Stan returned to the 3rd in time to participate in a raid on the German trenches at Richecourt on the night of May 30. He now had an assistant surgeon and decided to leave him to receive the wounded. Stan went with the troops, "for the value of the experience," as he explained, and also to treat casualties if the attackers were cut off by a German barrage to their rear. Between two and three in the morning of May 31 he saw the starlit valley between the lines begin to fill with a dense, drifting mist that clung close to the ground; the gas had a "sweetish pungent odor somewhat like banana oil."

Some men, though slow to don their masks, returned from the raid feeling nothing worse than a burning sensation in their throats and tightness across the chest. They slept what remained of the night and woke short of breath, giddy, with elevated pulse-rate. The first case Stan saw was gasping for breath while a frothy pink fluid came from his mouth. He was undergoing one of the least-pleasant deaths ever devised by unmerciful humanity, slowly drowning as his own body fluids filled his damaged lungs. Within two days, the 3rd Battalion evacuated

19. Bayne-Jones to Surgeon, 101st Infantry, May 1, 1918 (Report on Trench Foot in 2nd Battalion 101st Infantry), and Bayne-Jones to Surgeon, 101st Infantry, May 1, 1918 (Sanitary Report on Seicheprey Sector), both in B-18, Box 9, SBJC. On the state of American preventive medicine, see Weston P. Chamberlain and Frank W. Weed, *The Medical Department of the United States Army in the World War: Sanitation* (Washington, 1926), VI, and Joseph F. Siler, *The Medical Department of the United States Army in the World War: Communicable Diseases* (Washington, 1928), IX.

225 men with phosgene poisoning. Apparently, an American high-explosive shell had fallen on a German ammunition dump, releasing the phosgene stored there—all in all, an unlucky venture by green troops.[20]

Stan was on the line continuously from April Fool's Day to May 15. By now an accomplished survivor, he got out of target areas just as shells started to fall, or got in just as they stopped. He was strafed by a German plane but escaped injury: "When you realize that the bullets are going beyond you—the exhibition seems *lovely*—the bullets sound like picking the three top strings of a harp—and the tracer-bullets on fire look like fireflies in the evening—." He watched spring come to the Western Front: a few still-living fruit trees burst faithfully into bloom; the endless rain was no longer unbearably cold. "The season is lovely and tender in spite of the war."

His courage and devotion began to win recognition. The British awarded him the Military Cross, their third highest decoration, for his work with the B.E.F.; he was mentioned in 26th Division orders. Wearing a newly sprouted mustache, he was made regimental surgeon of the 103rd Infantry, in line for a major's rank. But though his luck held, the war was going on too long. Shells got on his nerves as never before, and he thought of death: "You never know when the noise and iron are going to drive your spirit out to the quieter fields above the balloons and aeroplanes."[21]

In July, 1918, the 26th Division shifted from the Toul Sector to the Marne. The men rode in steel freight cars whose floors had been made comfortable with straw, gazing through the open doors at *La Belle France*. People on the roads stopped and waved to them, and village children flocked to the tracks, crying, "Biscuit, biscuit." They meant the two-inch-square hardtack crackers, and the soldiers threw them out

---

20. Medical Arrangements for Raid by 3rd Battalion, 101st U.S. Infantry, May 30–31, 1918, in B-19, Box 9, SBJC. See also reports for May 30–June 2, 1918, *ibid*. Overall, gas was a painful and distressing, but not particularly effective, weapon, except against ill-trained or unprepared troops. See *Defensive Measures Against Gas Attacks* (Headquarters, AEF, 1917), in B-24, Box 10, SBJC.

21. Bayne-Jones to Tante E, May 15 and May 30, 1918, in B-3, Box 8, SBJC.

by handfuls and the children scrambled for them. When his unit arrived, Stan embarked upon a civilian practice, the only one he ever
had, among the children of Lorraine. They reminded him of pictures in
old French songbooks at home, "appealing bright little people" in a
landscape of old gray villages and summer fields.[22]

He knew that something big was in preparation. Americans were
being summoned in growing numbers to aid the Allies' great counter-
offensive in the Aisne-Marne region. Stan's own sector had been won
only a few weeks before; the ground was littered with excrement, dead
horses, dead men; flies swarmed and droned in the heat. The men endured "the most prolonged distresses—bombardments, gas at night."

The 26th Division went on the attack against a German salient
between Rheims and Soissons. The line of advance covered Torcy, Belleau, Givry, the Bouresche Woods, and Point 190 overlooking Chateau-
Thierry. Near Belleau Wood the soldiers advanced across wheatfields
in the face of machineguns. They rested among shattered trees, under
a chilly rain. But they felt they were winning, and Stan shared their
exultation. "Perhaps I will be able to remember the details as well as
the glory of it—when I get back," he wrote. On July 30, he sent George
Denegre a telegram that said simply, "Well great days."[23]

On leave from the front he had a spree in Paris, splurging $200.
But when he returned to his new regiment, resting and training in the
Côte d'Or, he had more than a hangover: he had caught "the grippe,
which takes away interest in life." The so-called Spanish influenza had
appeared in the United States during the spring and may have crossed
the ocean with American troops. A second and more severe wave would
follow in the autumn; during September and October it would cause
3,000 to 9,000 cases a week among the AEF, and the death rate in the
pneumonia that was often its sequel would surpass forty-five percent.

22. Bayne-Jones to Marian, June 2, 1918, *ibid.*

23. Bayne-Jones to Tante E, July 2 and July 15, 1918, and to Marian, July 28, 1918,
all *ibid.* Telegram, Bayne-Jones to Jeorge Denegre, Neworleans [*sic*], in B-21, Box 9, SBJC.
For objective accounts of the successive St. Mihiel and Meuse-Argonne offensives, see Edward M. Coffman, *The War to End All Wars: The American Military Experience in World
War I* (New York, 1968), 262–84, 300–348, and Allan R. Millett and Peter Maslowski, *For
the Common Defense: A Military History of the United States of America* (New York, 1984),
354–60. See also American Battle Monuments Commission, *26th Division: Summary of Operations in the World War* (Washington, 1944), 8, 21.

In all, some 550,000 Americans and more than 21 million people world-wide would perish, victims of a viral disease that medicine as yet could neither prevent nor cure.

Even as the great pandemic spread, the Allies won victory after victory, pressing a weary though not broken foe. In long night marches the 103rd returned to the line. The 26th Division pushed into the St. Mihiel Salient near Les Eparges, a region fought over since 1914—trenches, craters, barbed wire tangles hundreds of yards long—in persistent rain and through heartbreaking mud. Going over the top at 5 A.M. on September 12, the Americans worked their way through passages cut in their own wire toward gaps blown in the enemy's. They passed over the first German line with little difficulty, unaware that their foes were withdrawing before them.

But at the second, heavy machine-gun fire began to arc blindly through the dense, rainy darkness. The infantry worked around the nests and killed or captured the gunners one by one. The penetration of the salient rapidly deepened. As morning broke the Americans freed French villages on the anniversary of their capture four years before. Stan watched weeping civilians "[fall] on the necks of our men." At dark on the 13th they reached their objective, St. Maurice, and—liberating German stores, including beer—drank and feasted amid the blaze of homes and churches fired by the retreating foe. "Nothing will stop us—now," Stan exulted, writing from a shack in the woods, somewhere on the Woevre plain with its hundreds of smoldering fires.[24]

By now his own work was thoroughly professional. He set up his advanced aid stations and distributed his litterbearers and supplies, personally guiding them to the collection points. He kept track of problems in evacuation as they developed, and they were many: traffic blocked the roads; the litterbearers, obstructed by craters and wire, could not cross the worst spots in the line; ambulances bogged down,

24. Bayne-Jones to Uncle George, August 10 and September 2, 1918, and to Tante E, September 16, 1918, all in B-3, Box 8, SBJC. See also Regimental Intelligence and Operations Officer, 103rd Infantry, to C/S [Chief of Staff], 26th Division, September 19, 1918, Report of Action 12th September–14th September 1918 in St. Mihiel Salient, in B-22, Box 9, SBJC. On the flu epidemic, see *Weekly Bulletin of Disease*, No. 28 (October 21, 1918), 1, in Box 3309, RG 120, NARA; Alfred W. Crosby, *Epidemic and Peace, 1918* (Westport, Conn., 1976), 25, 207. The action that Bayne-Jones saw as a triumph was in reality a diversionary attack. See Harry A. Benwell, *History of the Yankee Division* (Boston, 1919), 173.

falling behind the advancing troops. Somehow Stan kept everything moving, extracting his 159 wounded from the tangle behind an American victory that was later to be judged comparatively easy.[25]

Stan was a veteran several times over and looked the part. Lice and red fleas swarmed on him, and he scratched incessantly. When the Meuse-Argonne offensive got under way, he lived in woods, shacks, and German dugouts, following a slow, bloody, difficult American advance. His only uniform was torn, snagged on barbed wire, frayed at the cuffs, one elbow worn through. When he sat down on a wet plank, "something tells me that there is a bald spot in the seat of my trousers."[26]

Long fought over, the region was a nightmare. Rotting German field boots still held leg bones. Fog and rain lowered on the torn earth, scattered with broken skulls, old green cartridges, decaying belts, rusting rifle barrels, tin cans, and the refuse of the trenches. Stan had much work to do: the Americans paid for their victory with a decimated First Army, contributing their own dead to the old battlefield.

Fighting continued to the very last days. Yet the Germans, facing a new war with a new enemy at the end of four exhausting years, had but a bleak future. On October 17, 1918, the German emperor accepted the resignation of his chancellor, and Field Marshal von Hindenburg gave assurance that the army would approve peace overtures. On November 8, the 26th Division saw positive evidence of a break, as the enemy began to retreat before them. They followed to Flabas and a "nasty bit of woods" to the east called the Bois de Ville. Diplomats agreed on a day and time for an armistice, but no one could be sure what would happen. At Flabas the Americans attacked again and were still in motion up to the stroke of eleven o'clock in the morning of November 11 when, Stan wrote, "all the game stopped."

He knew the time of day by the sudden silence. He was picking his way down a ravine, leading a party of litterbearers toward a wounded man, when a machine gun opened up and the bullets came clipping by. They fell on their bellies—and suddenly the war was over.

25. Report on Medical Service, 103rd Infantry in action of September 11–14, 1918 (Battle of San Mihiel Salient), September 22, 1918, in B-22, Box 9, SBJC.
26. Bayne-Jones to Aunt Susie, September 27, 1918, in B-3, Box 8, SBJC.

The machine gun ceased fire. The last German "freight car" rattled overhead. All the guns fell silent. In the cold, dense mist that hung over the battlefield Stan could hear water dripping from a bush. It was all "mysterious, queer, unbelievable." The men sat up, turned to their neighbors, asking if it were really over. Someone's voice said, "I guess I'll go look for some grub."

As the day wore on, the soldiers began to feel livelier. By nightfall the front had turned into a celebration. "Our men and the Boches are shooting up all the flares and rockets in the [ammunition] dumps." Along the lines thousands of lights blazed and dimmed, green stars, red stars, golden rain, all the signals that once had called for a barrage or warned of an attack. Now the rockets went up by the hundreds and nothing followed but rejoicing. From a hillock Stan watched the "strangest sight of the war," as a line of little fires spread along the American line, and not far off, another along the German. No longer afraid of a bullet, men were warming themselves against the autumn cold.[27]

For a few days they lay in the desolate country, holding what was called Neptune Sector, from Beaumont to Flabas. Then the men of the 26th Division gathered their gear and hiked 110 miles, to Chauffort near Langres. Along the way things important and unimportant happened to Stan. At Bazoilles—Base Willie to the Americans—he visited Base Hospital No. 18, the Johns Hopkins unit. His future wife happened to be there, but he did not meet her. He got a bath and clean underwear and bought himself a secondhand uniform to replace the tatters he wore. He passed his thirtieth birthday. On November 14 he was promoted to major, medical corps. And he learned that a friend in the Hopkins unit had died of influenza, one victim among many in the lethal autumn outbreaks.

Assigned to division headquarters as sanitary inspector, he rediscovered comfort, with a room of his own, a limousine at his call,

27. Bayne-Jones to Tante E, November 26, 1918, and to Marian, November 11, 1918, both in B-4, Box 8, SBJC.

and lovely views of the countryside—checkered fields, white poplar-bordered roads—from "a quaint old town on a hill." Montigny-le-roi was built of soft gray stone walls and red tile roofs; it held a small American base hospital, an old church, a Hotel de Ville with a town clock that struck each hour twice, and six hundred or so inhabitants plus the American soldiers. Here, early in December, as the sun broke through the mist and the American and French flags were paraded side by side, Stan received the Croix de Guerre with a gold star. And here, at a French hospital, he and the other officers of the 26th Division shared Christmas dinner with President Woodrow Wilson, come to participate in the peace conference.[28]

In January, 1919, he was ordered to Third Army headquarters as sanitary inspector of the army of occupation at Coblenz on the Rhine. In a letter, Stan reminded Marian of their travels before the war, when they had passed the town on the *Rheindampferschiff:* "That was in 1908 when we were young and vexed with being educated." A touristy, Kurortish place whose principal product was the wine grape, Coblenz boasted a cathedral with twin towers, a pompous memorial to Kaiser Wilhelm at the water's edge, and tree-lined drives along the Rhine and the Moselle. From Ehrenbreitstein—an old fortress rebuilt in the nineteenth century—panoramic views stretched away in a shimmer of winter mist or spring haze.[29]

For the conquerors, amenities and boredom marked their stay. They occupied the Grand Hotel Bellevue Coblenzer-Hof (a name that in itself evoked the whole prewar scene) and the wings of the *Schloss*, or palace. The occupation authorities informally licensed several brothels, and soon lines hundreds of men long formed outside. Among the officers much time was given to drinking, dancing, horseback riding, and casual venery. Among the ten officers in the Third Army's Office of the Chief Surgeon, a parody of the official health reports noted 10 cases of "nostalgia" and 9 of dipsomania; 199 prophylactic treatments; and an

28. Undated clipping, prob. New York *Times,* in B-33, Box 11, SBJC; Bayne-Jones to Tante E, December 15, 1918, in B-4, Box 8, *ibid.* See also Field Orders No. 118, 26th Division, December 16, 1918, and Letter, C/S to Officers, subject: Dinner for President, December 23, 1918, both in B-24, Box 10, *ibid.*

29. Bayne-Jones to Marian, January 16, 1919, in B-4, Box 8, *ibid.* See also *City of Coblenz and Environs* (GHQ-AEF, General Staff, n.p., n.d.), 11–20, in B-30, Misc. I, Box 11, *ibid.*

epidemic of swollen testicles caused by interposing one or both of those sensitive organs between the pommel and the rider's buttocks.

The Officers' Club was the local casino, and here Stan attended farewell parties for lucky comrades ordered home. But things were not always so amusing: the winter wave of the flu epidemic hit the army of occupation hard. Between January and March, 1919, more than 31,000 men were hospitalized for sickness, of whom about 13,000 suffered from "acute respiratory infections," mostly influenza. Ninety percent of the 664 deaths recorded in the first three months of the year were due to the pandemic, and against the disease there was little that the sanitary officer could do. It was no way to end a victorious war. Stan tracked the sicknesses of the region on a big wall map, noting that the flu was principally among the troops, typhoid among the civilians. [30]

Homesickness grew upon him. During the war Stan had used his connections to get into the fighting; now he used them to get away from the tedious life of the peacetime army. Uncle George communicated his plea for relief to Welch and Gorgas. Retired from the Army, but still rich in honor and influence, Gorgas contacted the new surgeon general, Merritte M. Ireland, former chief surgeon of the AEF, who wrote to his successor in Europe requesting Stan's release. After some delay, the chief surgeon of the Third Army called Stan in and dismissed him with seven words: "Goodbye, Major. You haven't been any trouble."

Stan landed at Newport News, Virginia, "feeling well," on May 28, 1919. Last of the three nations he had served, his own awarded him the Silver Star with two oakleaf clusters for gallantry under fire. A few days later he was discharged honorably at Camp Dix, New Jersey. [31] Besides his hard-earned decorations he carried away with him a grasp of wartime medicine that he could have gained in no other way, an acquaintance with preventive medicine at the most elementary level, and an assurance of his own courage and competence under stress.

30. Weekly Health "Bull," Hindquarters Third Base Army, Office of the Chief Sturgeon; Menu dated March 21, 1919; theater programs dated January 15 and 18, [1919], in B-31, Misc. II, Box 11, and ticket stubs and dance cards, various dates, in B-32, Misc. II, all in SBJC. On the epidemic, see Grissinger, *Medical Field Service*, 139, and Charles Terry Butler, *A Civilian in Uniform*, (N.p., 1975), 333. On brothels at Coblenz, see Phillips interview, 174.

31. Bayne-Jones to George Denegre, March 19, 1919, and May 28, 1919, from Red Cross Information Service at Newport News, Va., both in B-4, Box 8, SBJC.

As events would show, his life would be changed in consequence. But for the moment his thoughts were elsewhere; he felt a profound need for all the things that war had denied him, and he sought a laboratory, a career, and a wife.

FIVE

The Birth of a Career

The summer of 1919 was hot and troubled. The country was in a post-war depression, the attorney general was arresting and exiling Reds with scant regard for the Constitution, and terrorist bombs were going off in Washington and elsewhere. The Johns Hopkins Board of Trustees, meeting on June 3, 1919, voted Stan a one-year appointment as associate in bacteriology. But he lived in emotional doldrums. For him the excitement was over, and as far as his private life went, the war had settled nothing after all.

He found rooms on St. Paul Street about a block from his original quarters of 1911. As then, he felt "a stranger in a lonely town," and a beginner in medicine as well, his old, well-practiced skills gone rusty. Directing the laboratory was Professor of Pathology William G. Mac-Callum, a "rather sharp, critical man" who treated him as a stranger. Stan felt distant from everything, and he saw a similar loss of direction among others who had returned from the war.[1]

For a time he went about, gathering up boxes of books and other possessions he had left behind him, and tried to gather up his life, too. In the laboratory on the fifth floor of the pathology building his fingers slowly regained their cunning. He began to be able to make uncontaminated cultures again and felt that "things are coming around." The elemental fascination with the nature of life returned. "You can dish up life with a platinum loop," he was to say about the bacteriological laboratory. "It thrills you very much to think of that and to wonder what it is you're dealing with."[2]

1. Phillips interview, 180. MacCallum had distinguished accomplishments behind him but little ahead. A somewhat withdrawn, troubled man, his behavior indicated that "contradictory emotional forces were . . . at play" (A. R. Rich, "Dr. William George MacCallum, 1874–1944," *Bulletin of the Johns Hopkins Hospital*, LXXV [1944], 78).

2. Bayne-Jones to Marian, August 29, 1919, in B-38(1), Box 11, SBJC; Phillips interview, 190, 201. Laboratory workers use a loop of platinum wire to transfer bacteria from the petrie dish where they grow to a microscope slide for observation. "Contamination"—mixing different organisms in a culture—prevents the investigator from telling which ones produce the effects that he observes.

Despite a heavy teaching load—his first class had ninety students, a serious burden—Stan found time to do work of his own again. He remained an eclectic researcher, shifting from subject to subject as interest and opportunity directed. In this he followed both Welch and Zinsser, whose varied contributions to medical knowledge suggested the questing hound rather than the stalking, single-minded cat. And the teaching was by no means without interest. Abominating rote learning, Stan adopted a Socratic approach, asking questions calculated to set the students to teaching one another. "The students give the lecture," he said, "if you manage the class with tact and know when to put in the right word."[3]

But he felt a new loneliness rooted in the knowledge, recently discovered, of his real need for people. Previously he had seemed able to take the human race or leave it, sometimes charming everyone and sometimes withdrawing to his laboratory refuge. Life in the trenches had taught him a more elemental truth. "I do like people since the war as I should have liked them before," he told Marian in one of a sheaf of letters he wrote her to fill the gaps in his life. "Not getting to know them was my fault, though the reasons go very deep."[4]

He was almost thirty-one, and he knew what he needed. "I've been so introspective," he wrote her, "and had such thick blues since I've been back in this country that I'm worse than useless. Don't know exactly why—except possibly the need of that real companion you have advised me to find." Marian sent him a poem about magpies in Picardy, and he found himself thinking many times of the flight of birds, not as a scientist but "as poets or artists or lovers might: it fascinates the imagination." He was preoccupied with his unsatisfactory life, with sexual yearning and the flight of time.[5]

Recovering his normal verve was a slow process. That November he went riding at a friend's estate in brilliant fall woods; he celebrated his thirty-first birthday; he was elected to active membership in the Society of American Bacteriologists. He resumed the sociable ways he

3. Phillips interview, 215.
4. Bayne-Jones to Marian, September 14, 1919, in B-38(1), Box 11, SBJC.
5. Bayne-Jones to Marian, September 24, 1919, ibid.

had once known so well, though at dances he found the management of his feet difficult: "the ways of joy are laborious."[6]

Yet inwardly he remained an unhappy man. In January his laboratory burned down, set on fire by the explosion of a hydrogen-ion generator he had built himself. He put in three weeks of labor as hard as any he had known at Hopkins, moving the surviving equipment and setting it up again. As he worked with the pipefitters he received good tidings from New Orleans that served only to remind him of his loneliness. Marian again became a mother and Bayne and Alma were parents of a husky son. "I can think of hardly anything else," he wrote one of the new parents, "than that I wish I were in the place of either of you in that respect."

In June he was made an associate professor but only worried over the promotion; he felt that he did not deserve it, knew very little bacteriology, and had not accomplished anything in the year he had been home. He fretted that physical decay, or what passes for it at thirty-one, had set in. "I know that I am getting bald; a fly bit me right on the middle of the top of my head!"[7]

At last the fall of 1920 brought change. Stan loved to sail and to have young ladies accompany him. With two of them—Nannie Moore Smith, an X-ray technician at Hopkins, and her sister May—he bought a boat, a thirty-two-foot cabin sloop. His friendship with Nan grew quietly, in long days on the Chesapeake. Her life and his turned out to be curiously interwoven; a great-uncle with whom she lived had been a friend and classmate of Stan's grandfather, Thomas Levingston Bayne. Stan had just missed meeting Nan in France during the war, when she had served with the Johns Hopkins hospital unit at Bazoilles.

She was a woman of presence and force, with a taste for hard work that Stan liked, for it matched his own. Thirty years old, at five-foot-nine exactly as tall as he, Nan was a handsome woman but in some ways an odd one. Assertive and blunt-spoken beyond the custom of the time,

6. Bayne-Jones to Marian, November 13, 1919, and January 20, 1920, in B-38(2), Box 11, *ibid.*

7. Bayne-Jones to Marian, January 30, 1920, *ibid.*; Bayne-Jones to Marian, February 27, 1920, June 28, 1920, in B-38(3), Box 11, *ibid.* See also Phillips interview, 177, 182, 191–92.

she lacked one of his most evident qualities, a sense of humor. Many years later, a friend described her as "teacher-like"—big, solemn, intelligent, kind, and authoritative. She, too, felt the flight of time and hid demanding emotions beneath a controlled exterior.[8]

In due time, as his father had, Stan performed the Victorian ritual of asking for her guardian's consent to her marriage. The wedding preparations began in Baltimore amid a flurry of familial activity. Tante E and Uncle George arrived; Marian sent a rug that was too grand for the Bayne-Jones' small new apartment. But amid the happy confusion tragic news came from Philadelphia. With license and wedding ring in hand and ten days to wait for the ceremony, Stan had to rush to Aunt Susie Jones's bedside. Her appendix had ruptured. She survived the operation that followed but, as usual in the days before antibiotics, quickly developed peritonitis and septicemia. When Stan reached her, he found her unconscious; she died about an hour later.

So vanished another link to the old days, his onetime substitute mother perishing of a general infection as his natural mother had. Stan returned to Baltimore, and married Nan on June 25, 1921.[9]

For a time peace reigned. Stan wrote few letters, for he no longer needed to seek companionship by mail. His rare notes to Marian mirrored the world of a comfortable, youngish couple of domestic tastes. Stan took to pipe smoking and, like millions of Americans, responded to Prohibition by becoming a home brewer. He used a supply of Loewenbrau dry yeast that H. L. Mencken had obtained and Max Broedel had stored in his laboratory; his scientific skills came into play, and soon Stan was able to boast that "we . . . drink a beverage called beer which I can now make like a braumeister."[10] His wife rechristened him, beginning early in the marriage to call him B-J. Soon the name was adopted

8. Bayne-Jones to Marian, September 20, 1920, and January 22, 1921, both in B-38(3), Box 11, SBJC; Phillips interview, 218–19. Information on Nan's appearance and manner has been derived from lengthy conversations with people who knew her, especially an interview with Thomas Bayne and Louise Denegre, April 12–13, 1986, at White Stone, Va.
9. Bayne-Jones to Marian, June 15, 1921, in B-38(4), Box 11, SBJC.
10. Bayne-Jones to Marian, January 1, 1922, *ibid.* See also William Manchester, *H. L. Mencken: Disturber of the Peace* (New York, 1950), 169.

by everyone except his family and oldest friends. (And so this history will call him, from now on.)

The couple hoped for children but in this were disappointed. B-J promised his sister, "Someday,—we'll catch up—quadruplets twice or something like that." Instead, he had to be comforted by professional advancement. What came into the couple's lives during 1922 was not a child but a new job for B-J: quite a promising one.[11]

The offer came during the spring term from George H. Whipple. A student of Welch's, a teacher of B-J's, and a future Nobel laureate in medicine, Whipple was engaged in creating a new school of medicine at the University of Rochester in upstate New York. He was a quintessential New Englander, with the look of a shrewd and genial farmer, but he was to become a power in medicine. After seeing B-J at work in his laboratory, Whipple asked him to head the independent department of bacteriology he meant to establish.

Quickly, B-J visited Rochester and met the university president, Rush Rhees. He examined the plans and provisions for the new school and found them "inspiring." Inspiration was necessary, for as yet nothing else existed but a sandy field near a cemetery on the bank of the Genesee River. Money, however, was abundant. The General Education Board of the Rockefeller Foundation had embarked on a scheme to improve one medical school in each region of the country, so that competition would force the others to adopt reforms. Finding New York institutions slow to change, Abraham Flexner chose the University of Rochester as a promising place to build a first-rate school from scratch. He hoped for and later extracted millions from George Eastman, the Kodak king who was Rochester's leading citizen, to match the Rockefeller gift.[12]

By mid-October, B-J was ready to accept the challenge of pio-

11. Bayne-Jones to Marian, July 25, 1922, in B-38(4), Box 11, SBJC.

12. Bayne-Jones, "A Teacher by Preference," *Science*, CXLIII (January 24, 1964), 347; George H. Whipple, "Autobiographical Sketch," *Perspectives in Biology and Medicine*, II (Spring, 1959), 253–87; and George W. Corner, *George Hoyt Whipple and His Friends: The Life-Story of a Nobel Prize Pathologist* (Philadelphia, 1963). On Rochester's School of Medicine and Dentistry, see Abraham Flexner, *I Remember: The Autobiography of Abraham Flexner* (New York, 1940), 285–88, and Edmund Atwater, *et al.*, *To Each His Farthest Star* (Rochester, N.Y., 1975).

neering a new department in a new school. B-J could draw his own floor plans, choose many of his staff, and shape the style and spirit of the department and the school. His laboratory was not only to teach but to do the diagnostic work of the Rochester Health Bureau and two planned hospitals. As director of the health bureau laboratories, B-J could hire and fire city workers regardless of their politics. Soon the walls and tables in the Bayne-Jones apartment were covered with plans. "My shop will have 30,000 square feet of space," he reported with wonder. "It is a big opportunity and I get more excited over it the more I think about its possibilities." [13]

Meanwhile he needed to learn—and also to relax. Supported by Rochester, he took Nan to Europe during the summer of 1923. They visited London, Oxford, Edinburgh, and Brussels. At Paris, B-J formed a friendship with the French investigator Gaston Ramon, who taught him a method for gauging the strength of diphtheria toxin that B-J later introduced into American practice. Then, while Nan lingered west of the Rhine, he paid a quick visit to Berlin, stunned to find that a newspaper cost seven million marks; the inflation that ruined much of the German middle class was in full swing. At Stockholm's Karolinska Institute he encountered studies of bacterial variation that fascinated him; at a later time, he would pass on to American students the interest in mutation that was awakened here. From the sort of European pilgrimage that American doctors had been making for centuries, B-J returned, full of new ideas, to the utterly different world of upstate New York. [14]

He and Nan moved to Rochester early in 1924. The region differed from any that either had previously known. Though the city's style was provincial and its aspect somewhat dour, an unusual local culture had been shaped by industry and science since the days of the Erie Canal. The growth of Bausch and Lomb had made Rochester a center

13. Bayne-Jones to Marian, January 11, 1923, in B-38(5), Box 11, SBJC. Bayne-Jones benefitted from the innovations of George W. Goler, Rochester's public health chief, whom he always credited with combining city and university resources in this innovative way.
14. Bayne-Jones to Marian, June 24, July 21, and September 9, 1923, all in B-38(5), Box 11, SBJC; Phillips interview, 220–32. See also Bayne-Jones, "The Titration of Diphtheria Toxin and Antitoxin by Ramon's Flocculation Method," *Journal of Immunology*, IX (November, 1924), 481–504, and Bayne-Jones, *The Newer Knowledge of Bacteriology and Immunology* (Chicago, 1928), 759–71.

for the manufacture of fine lenses. In the 1880s, George Eastman had launched his remarkable photographic enterprise. Immensely successful, he had transformed the city by his philanthropy, building the Eastman School of Music, a technological institute, and a dental clinic. The concentration of specialized manufacturing with a scientific cast had given Rochester a robust intellectual and artistic life.

Such amenities helped to soften the shock of the bitter winter weather that sealed the windows of the Bayne-Joneses' new home with ice. Nan formed acquaintanceships among the university ladies. B-J found the people civic-minded, hospitable and—like New Orleanians—clubby. He joined the local medical society and enjoyed the local musical productions (though *Faust* sung in English left him politely skeptical). Because Whipple devoted all possible time to his laboratory, B-J, like the other faculty members, found himself taking on added duties as the school's ambassador to the Rochestrians, a part he relished and, with his diplomatic skill, played well.

His letters portrayed a quiet home, an absorbing job. Nan played the piano, and they bought in Rochester a new grand with a "wonderful, rich tone." Through the year, the immense building that was to house the medical school and both hospitals grew; B-J hoped that by the time another winter began he would be in his new laboratory.[15]

Here all was promise and confusion. The tastes of both Eastman and Whipple tended toward spareness, and in consequence the medical school belonged to what the philanthropist called the early penitentiary style of architecture. Unplastered, sanded brick walls predominated; the bare cement floors were sealed with linseed oil; the pipes were left exposed.

All the money went for equipment and room to work. Many of the faculty were young. In the early days, when the department stood unfinished, none of the partitions up, it looked "as big as several drill halls." A visiting German biologist was introduced to the new faculty

15. Bayne-Jones to Marian, January 20, 1925, in B-44, Box 12, SBJC. See also Bayne-Jones to "Good-Looking-Flapper-Mother-of-Five" [Marian], February 10, 1924, and to Marian, October 4, 1924, and August 9, 1925, all *ibid.* See also Phillips interview, 236–37.

and given a tour. He pointed to the vast open space, and said: "From zere to zere it is about one-fifth of a mile. Ze professors, no beards. Zis is a barn and all ze professors are boys."[16]

Whipple also followed his New Hampshire upbringing in the tight rein he kept on expenditures. Stan learned that if he wished to buy even test tubes for his laboratory, the dean must approve. Soon the pressure bred a revolutionary spirit among the department heads; they met secretly on the enclosed fire stairs and plotted an attack on Whipple in President Rhees's presence at some future meeting of the advisory board. But the president, catching wind of the plans, headed off the blowup. He called the cabal together and asked if they had any suggestions for relieving the dean's office of excessive administrative work. Somebody said at once, "Yes, give us control of our budgets." Rhees then spoke to Whipple, who wisely agreed. Understandably, B-J was to remember Rhees for the rest of his life as "one of the wisest educational administrators I ever met."[17]

The laboratory opened in 1925. Teaching was an art that B-J loved, and he gloried in the high quality of students, the small classes, and the fact that school, laboratories, and hospital were all under one roof. A student learning a particular disease could follow it from the microscope slide through the wards to the autopsy room. By establishing assistantships and fellowships with university backing, B-J attracted able young people from other universities; he drew into his laboratory other members of the medical school who were interested in bacteriology; he provided research opportunities for practicing physicians with scientific yearnings; and he brought to Rochester a scattering of able people from abroad.[18]

As an executive, he supervised about thirty people in the department of bacteriology and another thirty-six in the Rochester Health Bureau laboratory. His secretary spoke of "our noisy, busy department," and wondered how B-J kept his patience when he "had a million interruptions all day, every day." To escape the throng, he started rising

16. Goler to Bayne-Jones, June 16, 1932, in B-48, Box 12, SBJC; see also Flexner, *I Remember*, 214. There is a variant of Goler's story in Corner, *George Hoyt Whipple*, 154.
17. Phillips interview, 258, 260, 256, 280–81.
18. *Ibid.*, 272.

at six and hastening to the laboratory, to get in a little work when no one else was around.[19]

In this way he added to his bibliography despite the pressures of teaching and administration. At Hopkins, since his return from the war, he had written mainly on immunology. At Rochester, his work led him, among many other topics, to spread knowledge of Ramon's methods in assessing the strength of diphtheria toxin and antitoxin, and—an improvement on earlier work that had aroused widespread interest—to experiment with the use of motion-picture film to obtain action microphotographs of bacterial growth. He was fortunate in finding an able physiologist to be his coauthor; Edward F. Adolph took measurements of bacterial growth from the pictures that B-J and an Eastman technician had made. As usual, B-J's near-dyslexia in handling figures hobbled his scientific work: "Don't trust my arithmetic," he cautioned Adolph: "As no sum in division, multiplication, subtraction or addition that I do ever comes out twice with the same answer, I am in a mess most of the time."[20]

Yet the laboratory work that he pursued despite all obstacles became steadily less important to him. If his talents drew him toward administration, his failings pushed him in the same direction. Burdened as he was in handling mathematics, his achievements in the laboratory represented a triumph of determination and hard work over native mediocrity. He could win no distinction there. Since distinction was what he sought, he had to try something else.[21]

By contrast, his skills as an administrator were near-instinctive. His tact, decency, and fairness enabled a large, mixed staff of men and women, academics and state employees to work harmoniously and fruitfully together. He made the work of the health bureau his special concern. Though it was largely routine and at all seasons heavy, B-J

19. Creegan to Bayne-Jones, July 15, 1932, in B-51(1), Box 12, SBJC.

20. See notes accompanying Bayne-Jones to Adolph, August 14 and 30, 1932, in author's private collection. See also Bayne-Jones and C. Tuttle, "An Apparatus for Motion Picture Photomicrography of the Growth of Bacteria," *Journal of Bacteriology*, XIV (1927), 157–73; Bayne-Jones and Edward F. Adolph, "Growth in Size of Micro-Organisms Measured from Motion Pictures," *Journal of Cellular and Comparative Physiology*, I (June, 1932), 387–407, 409–27, and II (December, 1932), 329–48.

21. Phillips interview, 209.

early decided that it must take precedence, for patients demanded quick and accurate answers, a sense of urgency transmitted by their doctors to the laboratory. The Rochester police made its own pressing demands, expecting B-J to aid in murder cases by distinguishing between human and animal blood. "There is," B-J said later, "more than meets the eye in bacteriology."[22]

Under the pressure, he rediscovered the fundamental appeal of preventive medicine. Rochester's leader in public health was George W. Goler, an able and incorruptible man who fascinated B-J by his own abilities and by his resemblance to B-J's image of Joseph Jones. Like Jones, Goler faced down municipal politicians to protect his workers from the demands of patronage and the community from disease. B-J aided him by applying his own capacity for systematic work to the laboratory, where, with university and city backing, the staff increased and the number of examinations done yearly multiplied by six or seven times. "No one knows," said Goler, "what you have meant to us."[23]

More than local recognition came B-J's way. Soon he was in daily contact, professional or personal, with virtually all important centers of medical research. Much of his correspondence dealt with the swapping of microorganisms, for no national organization yet existed to maintain cultures of bacteria, fungi, and yeasts. Hence each laboratory kept its own microscopic zoo, begging what it needed from others and supplying others in turn. His spare time was taken up with meetings and papers. He joined the American Association of Immunologists and served as its president and as president of the Society of American Bacteriologists and the New York State Association of Public Health Laboratories. Such diverse honors reflected his widening interests. He taught the summer term of 1929 at the University of Chicago, where, under the influence of L. G. Taliaferro, he became interested in parasites. Taliaferro was an old friend and a leader in the field. Back in Rochester, B-J renamed his department Microbiology, to signal his concern with all the microscopic world.[24]

22. *Ibid.*, 247, 286–87.
23. Goler to Bayne-Jones, June 6, 1932, in B-48, Box 12, SBJC; see also Phillips interview, 207–08; Corner, *George Hoyt Whipple*, 134–37.
24. George Packer Berry to Bayne-Jones, February 25, 1932, in B-55(A–B), Box 13, SBJC; Phillips interview, 270–79.

He directed his habit of scholarship and interest in history critically upon his dual profession as doctor and bacteriologist, and spoke candidly to his colleagues about the conflicts and failures he perceived under the startling triumphs of the bacteriological era in medicine. Their specialty, he declared in his presidential address to the Society of American Bacteriologists, formed a mass of more or less accurate observations rather than a science with a coherent inner theory. Adding to its problems was its servitude to medicine. The doctor, concerned with diagnosis, was able through his dominance in hospitals and schools to impose his own demands upon his "bacteriological coolie," treating him as a worker who did tests to aid diagnosis, not as a colleague in a related science. In turn, the supposition that microbes caused infectious disease—in fact, they only formed a necessary element in causation—diverted doctors from the study of patients to the "supposedly specific microbe." The result of the marriage of bacteriology and medicine had been to impede the development both of a science of experimental medicine focused on the patient, and a science of bacteriology devoted to the study of the basic phenomena of life. The medical bacteriologist "yearns for the statement of a generalization which will satisfy many of the questions answered so superficially by the Koch-Pasteur germ theory of disease, and . . . repeats with crossed fingers the glib phrases of the functional jargon of immunology."[25]

B-J was not original in voicing such reservations. He was, however, performing a service for his colleagues that he was often to repeat in the future—that of putting basic questions to them from an unassailable position within the profession itself.

He traveled much and spoke often at scientific meetings. He received many visitors in his home, where he and Nan practiced a warm and unassuming hospitality. (During one five-month period, about 150 guests passed through the house, pausing for anything from a single meal to a lengthy stay.) A substantial part of his social life was academic

25. Bayne-Jones, "Reciprocal Effects of the Relationship of Bacteriology and Medicine," *Journal of Bacteriology*, XXI (1931), 61–73, 71, 67. The basic theory that Bayne-Jones demanded was not far away. See Foster, *History of Medical Bacteriology and Immunology*, 170–71; Boris Magasanik, "Research on Bacteria in the Mainstream of Biology," *Science*, CCXL (June 10, 1988), 1435–39.

and medical politicking, even though he sought no definite position. Yet his dealings with his colleagues revealed a natural generosity, an unpremeditated rightness in word and act. Whatever his ambitions, B-J was doing what came naturally, not playing a role. His ear was flawless for the tactful word, and he made sure of saying it, either in person or by handwritten note. Together, work and socializing absorbed his life and Nan's. [26]

Yet even as B-J made his mark in the professional world where he functioned so well, in his own home, behind the facade of hospitality, problems began to fester. In the late twenties the consequences almost destroyed his marriage.

In 1925 the Bayne-Joneses started to make yearly visits to Biloxi, renting a house near Malua. The children of summers past had become the adults, vacationing with their spouses—B-J and Nan, Marian and Ralph, Bayne and Alma. The children who splashed in the warm shallows or took their first sailing lessons were a new generation. Tante E remained much as she had always been, only stouter and, if possible, more formidable than in the past. Her arrivals were royal progresses, greeted with dread. She made herself mistress of the house, turned meals into stiff and formal Victorian repasts, and sewed costumes for amateur theatricals. She wrote the scripts herself and forced everyone to take part, whether they wished to or not. [27]

Despite Edith, Nan appeared to enjoy the clan as a whole. She liked her sisters-in-law, comparing them favorably with the people at Rochester where, it seemed, she was less happy than during the first year. "You and Alma," B-J wrote from the North to his sister, "are the kind of friends she needs, but doesn't find up here. These people never seem to become our own people." Attractions for both Bayne-Joneses were Marian's children. "I wish I could match him with one of my own," wrote B-J of a nephew and namesake. But Nan continued childless. [28]

26. See correspondence in B-55(A–B, C–E, and F–G), Box 13, SBJC.
27. Interview with Thomas Bayne and Louise Denegre.
28. Bayne-Jones to Marian, July 28 and November 23, 1925, and November 15, 1924, all in B-44, Box 12, SBJC.

And, it would seem, increasingly unhappy. "Nan has really been the one who has had the vexatious life," he wrote on one occasion, "as things have been difficult for her at times." If Nan felt isolated at Rochester, the reason can only be guessed from her later patterns of behavior. She had a downright way about her, and her blunt-spoken opinions, uncomfortably perceptive yet lacking the grace of humor, may have given offense. She possessed, as events were soon to show, a deep capacity for suspicion, and she was inwardly guarded, sociable and kind yet unable to make close friends.

She shared her husband's life only to a degree. B-J left the house early and did not return until late; he traveled frequently at a time when even a short trip could mean a week from home. The professional life that absorbed him excluded her. B-J transformed their parlor into a "complete library stack" of scientific books, and when his colleagues visited they talked science while she remained silent. Hospitality to students alleviated her loneliness; she gave them dinners, and her very solemnity endeared her to them, for she took them even more seriously than they took themselves. However, as many a wife has discovered, she could be sociable yet isolated, overworked but peripheral, busy about her husband's life yet without a life of her own.[29]

The relations of husband and wife may have shown other strains. B-J's genial exterior hid a sometimes rough determination to have his own way that was noted both by family members, who saw him off camera, and by subordinates, who found him an exacting taskmaster. The same willfulness must have surfaced at home. Hints of even more basic troubles sometimes emerged. When he married, B-J was sexually experienced, while his wife, liberated in word, may have been a puritan in deed. Echoes of his prewar love affair occasionally sounded in family correspondence. Recalling it, Tante E wrote encouragingly that "the war . . . I am sure blotted out many memories, & that love you brought Nan was pure intense & beautiful & I can't help hoping & believing that she will yet realize this."[30]

29. Bayne-Jones to Marian, November 23, 1925, in B-44, Box 12, SBJC; see also Bayne-Jones to Uncle George, March 18, 1928, in B-59 (Family), Box 13, *ibid*. See also author's interview with Adolph, May 2, 1986, Rochester, New York, in author's collection.

30. Tante E to Bayne-Jones, July 27, 1928, in GDC.

Nan did not appear to share these sentiments; she accused B-J of having indulged in an abnormal relationship rather than a merely unsuitable one. As relations deteriorated during 1927 and 1928, she began to speak bitterly of his character, writing to members of his family to denounce him and to state her case against him in terms that were, for the time, unusually graphic. Nan also accused her husband of being a failure, apparently on the grounds that they were unable to escape Rochester, which she had come to hate.[31]

Within B-J's family the facade of the marriage crumbled. The energetic and successful doctor, the hospitable and gracious wife, had in fact spent difficult years together. He was relieved to have Edith, George, and Bayne know the truth, acknowledging that "she and I have had very hard times since we were married. . . . I have realized that there is a great deal of truth in many of her criticisms and that her marriage to me has been a tragic time for her." Nan felt often that she could not abide his presence, while B-J lived from day to day, not sure whether she would stay or go, or what another season might bring.[32]

As to the real root of the trouble, Nan's failure to conceive may have explained much. Her relations with her husband steadily declined as the term of her childbearing years approached. "Knowing now her hypersensitiveness about the possibility that she may be blamed for not having children which is almost an obsession"—wrote Tante E, who understood such things—"I understand a little why she resented my letter feeling that I compared my case with hers." Nan needed children, if only to have a life of her own apart from that of her busy, often-absent husband. Failing to become pregnant (and that in a clan where babies were all but universal and obligatory), she projected upon him not only her sense of failure but her resentment of a marriage that both monopolized and excluded her.[33]

Of her real and agonizing distress there could be no doubt. She began to suffer from skin problems—hives, pruritus, urticaria, the name differs from letter to letter. B-J, who understood the weight of

31. Tante E to Bayne-Jones, August 18, 1928, and George Denegre to Bayne-Jones, September 3, 1928, both *ibid.*
32. See typescript copy of letter, Bayne-Jones to Tante E, August 21, 1928, *ibid.*
33. Tante E to Bayne-Jones, September 7, 1928, *ibid.*

words, described one attack as "torture." Baffled, he turned to specialist friends for advice. Nan tried one thing after another. In 1928 she
visited Johns Hopkins for treatment. At some point she had a tonsillec-
tomy (the cure-all of the time) and took an unspecified "intravenous
treatment" as well. A physician in Cooperstown, New York, recommended a medicine he had tried only once but with 100 percent success. "Unfortunately," wrote B-J in 1929, "we have started a dozen plans
of treatment with that hope [of cure], only to find ourselves deeply
disappointed at the end."[34]

At some point B-J's friends at Hopkins reached the conclusion that
Nan's "generalized pruritus involving large areas of the skin" was caused
by a "nervous condition believed to have arisen from dissension in the
family." Nan told Alma that "the result of my visit to Hopkins is that
the doctors there as well as the ones here [in Rochester] insist that I
must separate from B-J."

She saw her husband now with deep bitterness. She called him "a
sick child"; his family were "either completely ignorant of his real character and disposition, or else completely liars, working against me instead of with me. If I could get him back to Baltimore or, best of all, to
New Orleans, there might be some hope for us. I'd rather do anything
than leave him, but what else can I do?"[35]

She spent a terrible summer in 1929. By fall she seemed to be
doing better, perhaps because her decision had been taken. On Sunday
morning, September 13, she told B-J that she had decided to leave him.
On September 29, a few days after the first break in the stock market,
he gave her $1,000 to finance the separation. Then she fled to Washing-
ton. Members of the family visited her at B-J's request, but when they
urged her to return to him Nan was even more than commonly blunt
in her indictment of her husband.[36]

Unhappy B-J, who had learned to keep people at a distance with
geniality, wit, the objectivity of science, had by now lost all chance of

34. Bayne-Jones to Marian, March 17 and August 4, 1929, in B-44, Box 12, SBJC;
Homer F. Swift to Bayne-Jones, April 17, 1929, in B-57(S–T), Box 13, *ibid.* See also G. M.
Mackenzie to Bayne-Jones, April 28, 1929, B-57(M), Box 13, *ibid.*

35. Memorandum for Record, T. B. Turner, August 29, 1979, Nan to Alma, May 30,
1929, and June 2, 1930, all in Bayne-Jones File, AMC.

36. Bayne-Jones memorandum, undated [probably September 29, 1929], in GDC.

defending his privacy. Unable to be objective, unable to laugh, Nan proved herself a most forceful and difficult antagonist for the man who, in spite of everything, still loved and wanted her. Her pen poured out a stream of letters to members of the clan, including her husband, and they in turn showered her with assurances of love. Painful to the people involved, the situation appeared absurd or comic to onlookers.

Yet the separation, lasting about six months, brought the beginnings of reconciliation. The signs of irrationality disappeared, and with them the skin disease. Seemingly, during the time when Nan lived apart, an emotional process began by which she adopted her husband as her child, enveloping him with her powerful protective instincts and turning her capacity for deep suspicion against his real and supposed enemies. A measure of newfound sexual sophistication may have helped the healing process. "Things are going much better with B-J and me," she wrote her confidante, Alma, from Rochester in June, 1930, after she had returned home. "I got some wonderful advice from a Doctor in Baltimore about him. It sounded awful to me at first but it works amazingly well. I won't bother you with it now."[37]

Gradually the crisis receded into the past, fading as her childlessness became inevitable; fading, too, as B-J began to separate himself from Rochester, with all its reminders of the couple's time of troubles. In the fall of 1929 he received an offer of a professorship from the University of Chicago. More intriguing was a whisper that reached his ears in late 1930 or early 1931 of a possible opening at Yale.

Since the war his alma mater had been undergoing a rebirth as a new president, James R. Angell, aided by some remarkable deans, transformed a famous university into a great one. (The dean and rebuilder of the medical school was Milton C. Winternitz, the abrasive pathologist for whom B-J had worked at Hopkins before the war.) One of Angell's innovations was the residential college, designed to provide individual attention for upperclassmen and prevent learning from becoming, as it threatened to, a mere assembly line. Each college was to

37. Nan to Alma, June 2, 1930, in Bayne-Jones File, AMC.

have a master's house, dormitories, dining hall, recreation room, and library; the master and the faculty members who served as fellows were to provide counseling, discipline, and perhaps tutoring in academic subjects as well.

But Angell had another aim. He wished to see at least one college under a scientific man, to further the goal of integrating knowledge and to encourage the sort of interdisciplinary work that formed a cornerstone of his own policies at Yale. This goal, in the opinion of B-J's friends on campus, made B-J a suitable candidate.

In January, 1931, one such friend brought to Rochester the news that Angell wanted B-J. Deeply interested, he gave Angell a favorable reply but indicated that he wanted a laboratory of his own and an appointment as professor of bacteriology in the medical school as well. By the end of March, Angell had conceded everything, for Dean Winternitz—who had reasons of his own—had become an enthusiastic B-J supporter. On May 3, B-J and Nan visited New Haven, and by the end of the month all parties were in agreement. On June 6 he told Whipple that he would accept Yale's offer.[38]

That year the summer visits of the Bayne-Joneses to Malua, long interrupted during their troubles, resumed. Despite Tante E, whose capacity for self-dramatization had not been diminished by the recent death of George Denegre, B-J and Nan were able to rest, sail, and swim. Yet they seemed to love Bayne and Alma more than they did each other. The younger Denegres, with their thriving children enjoying the water and the sand, represented what the Bayne-Joneses had hoped to be, perhaps still blamed each other for not being. (B-J, during this stay at Biloxi, nicknamed his younger brother "Papa.")

When the summer ended, they left reluctantly for the North. They paused in Mobile, spending a hot night at the Battle House hotel. After dinner they sat silent in their room, "in nothing—B-J reading Time . . . and we having nothing but gloomy thoughts," wrote Nan to Alma. In a sad letter sprinkled with the word "nothing" as a leitmotiv,

---

38. Robert French to Bayne-Jones, January 29 and February [?], 1931, in C-24(1), Box 15, SBJC; see also Angell to Bayne-Jones, March 29, 1931, *ibid.* See also Winternitz to Carl A. Lohman, June 8, 1931, in James Rowland Angell Presidential Papers, Group No. 2-A-14, Acc. 12137, Box 183, SML.

she returned again and again to Alma's children, and to her own depression. "I really didn't think a person could be so low."[39]

B-J and Nan had been married for ten years, and would remain so for thirty-nine more—a curious passage for a marriage that evolved over time into one of those rare alliances whose partners seem to form one extraordinary being. In the end they would leave the achievements of B-J's life as common progeny. But for the time, in the hot hotel room at the end of summer, they were exhausted combatants, the battle ended but the nature of the peace to follow still unclear.

39. Nan to Alma, September 22, 1931, in Bayne-Jones File, AMC.

SIX

The First Triumph

During all his domestic troubles, B-J's career continued to rise. So firm was his reputation, so wide his acquaintanceship in the medical world, that it seemed to move by momentum even when the man himself was distracted or sick or weary. A turning point came during the time of transition between Rochester and Yale. B-J gained his first experience as a distributor of grant money, and he wrote two books that were successful in quite different ways.

The first was a small, readable volume that represented B-J's only attempt to enlighten the intelligent layman about his profession. In 1931 he was named a member of the science advisory board for a fair planned by the city of Chicago to alleviate the depression by creating jobs and bringing in visitors. Amid widespread poverty and want, the Chicago Century of Progress Exposition took form, burdened by a name either humorless or bitterly ironic. Science was a theme, and B-J agreed to contribute a popular account of bacteriology.

Man and Microbes used language simple to the point of transparency to celebrate the study of the invisible world. Microbiology, B-J held, was the "most liberating" of the sciences, offering ways to prevent or cure illness, but above all stripping disease of its dire mythology. "Man is nowadays conscious of opposing another living thing, a microbe, not an immaterial arrow of a god, not a ghostly horseman and not a poisonous wraith." Such wisdom emerged from the laboratory, whose ambience B-J rendered in one memorable sentence: "The microbiologist works in the midst of steam, blue gas flames, hot wires, cotton plugs, appetizing smells, foul odors, jewel-like lenses, bright spotlights, brilliant colors, patient animals, long words and the smallest specks of life."

Written in three weeks and sold for a dollar, the little book proved to be one of the more popular of the series put out for the fair, and won B-J a small sheaf of complimentary reviews as well. ("Voila de l'excellente vulgarisation," exclaimed a Paris newspaper.) Reconcilia-

tion at home may have been reflected in his dedication of the book
"To Nan."[1]

His second book was entirely different: a revision of Hans Zinsser's
standard textbook of bacteriology. The work began, curiously enough,
in a misunderstanding between old friends. During World War I, Zinsser, working for the Red Cross, had seen typhus at first hand in Serbia.
Later his research increasingly centered on the disease, especially on
the louse-borne epidemic form with its high mortality and traditional
associations with hunger, winter, and war. He wished to write a popular
book about typhus, allowing his natural lively style an outlet that scientific publications denied it.

But between his laboratory and his book, Zinsser lacked time to
revise his textbook, a complex task that had to be done periodically as
the science changed and grew. In 1927, at the request of the AMA's
Morris Fishbein, B-J reviewed the newly published sixth edition and
sent his essay to Zinsser for comment. Receiving no answer, B-J submitted his work to the *Journal of Infectious Diseases*, where it duly appeared, unsigned in accord with the magazine's policy of the time. Sparks
flew in consequence. No author—especially not the high-tempered
Zinsser—likes to be told that his book's multitude of errors will serve a
great end by emancipating students from the tyranny of the printed
page.

Returning from a stay in Algeria with Charles J. H. Nicolle—
discoverer of the fact that lice transmit typhus—Zinsser read the seemingly anonymous attack, penned an angry letter to his critic, and posted
it to the editor. B-J replied at once, reminding Zinsser of his earlier
offer, saying that he hoped the incident would not injure their friendship and that "whatever is wrong may be made right."

The reply was a burst of apology and candor about the textbook.
"I am a terrible old muddle-head, getting senile—probably because of
alcoholism," Zinsser said. Further: "The book revision was a careless

1. Stanhope Bayne-Jones, *Man and Microbes* (Baltimore, 1932), 120, 20; Review of
Man and Microbes in Paris *Journal de Debats*, June 30, 1932; Hugh A. Bayne to Bayne-
Jones, March 1, 1933, in C-2, Box 13, SBJC. Since Bayne-Jones wrote, religious interpreta-
tions of the AIDS epidemic have shown how far humankind is from giving up mystical theories
of disease.

job. During the time that I was doing it I was deep in filtration and allergy and, at night, in my literary dilletantisms." He admitted receiving other critical reviews. "Perhaps I ought to give up continuing [the textbook]. We'll see."[2]

At the end of 1930, B-J found himself in Boston for a professional meeting and stayed with Zinsser, now a fixture of Harvard's medical school. Amid the warm family atmosphere of his home, the two men rediscovered their mutual delight in convivial drinking, wide-ranging talk, and the laboratory. At some point Zinsser offered to make B-J coauthor of the textbook if he would undertake the lion's share of work on the next revision. For the moment B-J declined, but the idea remained with him. Perhaps he came to regret the missed opportunity. Ever a realist about his own abilities, B-J may have concluded that authorship of a text would exactly suit him. His lack of important original discoveries would not matter, and his encyclopedic grasp of his field, his clear prose, talent as a teacher, and seemingly boundless capacity for intelligent work could shine.[3]

One day when he was visiting his friend's laboratory at Harvard, he reversed himself and agreed to do the book. Once committed, he went at the project with his customary thoroughness. In the summer of 1932, skipping their customary visit to Biloxi, B-J and Nan spent about two months in New York City, where he labored in a monastic cell at the New York Academy of Medicine. Then they moved on to Washington, settling in Foggy Bottom in an apartment that overlooked the Potomac. Here B-J continued to work in the Surgeon General's Library, with a corner of his own in the stacks.

Yet the textbook was only a part of his reason for coming to Washington. He was also there to help distribute money to medical researchers. During World War I, the National Academy of Sciences, a semipublic body enjoying congressional patronage, had given birth to the National Research Council (NRC). By the thirties, the NRC sponsored

2. Bayne-Jones to Zinsser, September 21, 1927, Zinsser to Bayne-Jones, September 23, 1927, and "Thursday night," n.d., all in C-7(1), Box 14, SBJC. See also Bayne-Jones, MS Review of *A Textbook of Bacteriology*, by Hans Zinsser, M.D., *ibid.*

3. Bayne-Jones to Zinsser, January 10, 1931, and Zinsser to Bayne-Jones, January 13, 1931, both in C-7(2), Box 14, *ibid.*

conferences, awarded fellowships and grants, and acted as a planning and coordinating body for research in the natural sciences. Its *Bulletin* reported on the state of research throughout the country; its position as go-between for federal and private research interests was unique. Research-oriented physicians from the universities found a natural home in its medical-science division, now to be chaired by B-J for one year.[4]

Between the NRC and the textbook he carried a heavy burden. Yet he put his own stamp on the book, performing the primary work of updating the bulk of the text. "I think I wrote seven hundred thousand words in long hand," he said later, "which was a great labor." He feasted on hard-boiled eggs, trusting the mild indigestion they caused to keep him awake and upright. Zinsser contributed the section on immunology and chapters on tuberculosis, typhus, and encephalitis. Their contrasting personalities worked well together: B-J was cool, objective and thorough, Zinsser hard-driving, intuitive, and indifferent to small errors.

By the spring of 1933, B-J had the substance of the revised text in hand. The time when he would take up his duties at Yale was approaching as well. In April he visited New Haven, finding his fellows at Trumbull College "a pretty good lot of cultured ruffians," then passed on to Boston where he laid the manuscript on Zinsser's desk. Zinsser was delighted. The book was "100% better than it has ever been before," he exclaimed, and the reason was the "scholarly thoroughness" that B-J had brought to it.[5]

With his NRC experience and his name on a standard text, B-J was staking out a claim to a different kind of career from the one he had pursued hitherto. He had rejected the practitioner's office for the laboratory; now he had put aside the laboratory, too, as the place where he would spend most of his time and try to make his mark. But it remained unclear what Yale would mean to him, and whether his solid, unspectacular reputation as a medical scientist, teacher, and administrator would be enhanced or smothered by the university's demands.

4. Zinsser to Bayne-Jones, June 19, 1931, *ibid.*; see also Richard H. Shryock, *American Medical Research Past and Present* (1947; rpr., New York, 1980), 262–63, and Phillips interview, 306–09.

5. Phillips interview, 313; Zinsser to Bayne-Jones, April 24 and October 16, 1933, in C-7(4), and Zinsser to Bayne-Jones, October 19, 1933, in C-7(6), Box 14, SBJC.

As the textbook began its long trek through Appleton toward publication, B-J and Nan moved into the newly completed master's house of Trumbull College. Nan disliked its "girder-gothic" style (as a friend called it), and the site was noisy, bounded by three city streets, one with a trolley line. Yet Trumbull proved to have its charms. Though the master's house stood close to the dorms, the architect had foresightedly concentrated halls, stairways, closets, and pantries on that side, while the rooms the family lived in faced west toward the college courtyard, with a view of the huge library tower.[6]

Rebuilt by Angell, the Yale of B-J's student days had been transformed into a loving, detailed, often witty pastiche of medieval forms. Arches, stained-glass windows, quaint carvings, quiet courtyards, and walls of dense stone sheltered learning at the cost of separating it from the world outside, in a theatrical illusion of another time and place. And the university had changed in more than architecture.

In times past it had been a finishing school for young men of good family, its proudest product the "Yale man." Since then a new rigor had come to the campus and a new cynicism as well. Veterans disillusioned by the aftermath of their sacrifices in World War I had transmitted their feelings to their sons. The depression, now in its fifth year, had completed an upheaval in the outlook of the young. Fascism and communism both stirred interest. Students read the works of biographers whose pleasure lay in debunking the great. "Poor Shelley!" exclaimed Zinsser, who saw the same world from his post at Harvard. "Poor Byron! Poor Wagner! . . . And even poor Jesus!"

More soberly, B-J noted that "law was losing some of its sanctity," that criticism of all institutions was possible and even demanded. Sustaining the rebellious mood was a new and personal acquaintance with want. The students at Trumbull, a "cross-section of Yale," were by no means all the pampered sons of rich men. Many worked to earn their keep and some lived close to the edge of destitution.[7]

Yet they contrived to remain young. In the dormitories, the inevitable pipe-smoker stoked his engine with "rug-ravellings"; a practical

6. French to Bayne-Jones, August 9, 1931 in C-24(2), Box 15, *ibid.*
7. "[Letter from] Dr. Bayne-Jones," *15th Anniversary Trumbullian*, XV [1948?], 9, in C-29, Box 15, *ibid.*; Hans Zinsser, *Rats, Lice and History* (Boston, 1935), 5.

joker made the courtyard ring at three in the morning with cannon-crackers thrown from his window; winter brought "snow battles and windows broken." In the *Trumbullian*, the college paper, a column called "Dials and Discs" reviewed radio shows and the latest swing records. Absorbing preoccupations were girls, problems with money and transport, movies, and sunbaths on the eighteen-inch ledges of the dorms. Into this milieu B-J and Nan moved as counselors, social directors, and parent substitutes.[8]

One hundred and sixty-one young men shared Trumbull with the Bayne-Joneses. On Thursday evenings B-J and Nan held open house. Dances drew crowds; intramural sports and debates won passionate followings; a Trumbull Orchestra took form; and an International Affairs Group met every Wednesday evening for food sauced with pacifism. The dining hall, in B-J's opinion, was the actual heart of Trumbull, given the appetites of the young and the constraints that the depression placed on their wallets.[9]

A conscientious if often distracted master, B-J was available to the students at any hour when they could find him home. Working at night in the master's office, he would often hear a tap on the leaded panes of the window and admit a student who wished to talk. Sitting until the early hours, he heard "very astonishing case histories of young people growing up." Parents and love affairs, want of money and the pressure to succeed formed the burden of most tales, but as a doctor B-J heard about physical problems and family histories of illness as well. When the students departed into the workaday world, he wrote them fair, upbeat letters of recommendation.[10]

Though far from permissive in any doctrinaire sense, B-J resolved from the beginning to allow his charges to regulate their own lives as much as possible. Since the point of college was the entry into adulthood, he refused to perpetuate the preparatory-school system into university life. His censorship of the newspaper was, by his own description, loose. No proctors supervised the dorms, which were largely

8. "Trumbull Papers," *The Trumbullian*, I (January, 1934), 8, 9.
9. Bayne-Jones, "The First Quarter-Year," *The Trumbullian*, I (January, 1934), 5, 9–10, 11, 16, in C-32, Box 16, SBJC.
10. Phillips interview, 346, 354.

self-regulating; sophomores, juniors, and seniors all lived together and all three were unlikely to be going through the same phase at the same time.[11]

But B-J relied above all upon Nan. As his work for Yale expanded, she became more and more the unofficial headmistress of the college. Her social duties were onerous. The usual circuit of faculty get-togethers, a steady stream of visitors, and the needs of the college made a time-filling combination. But the students were her chief concern. The woman who had almost destroyed her marriage through her resentment of her childless state now lived a life that was saturated in youth. She counseled the Trumbullians with her customary intelligence, solemnity, and downright language, and displayed to advantage a royal memory that recorded names on first hearing. "Sometimes there would be fifty [students] in the Master's parlor," B-J recalled, "and she'd introduce everybody. I don't see how she did it, but it was wonderful." At any time from 1933 to 1939 Nan could have said, with Mr. Chips, that she had hundreds of children. She could not have said, as he did, that they were all boys, for the Master's house often bulged with the students' weekend dates, and Nan played chaperone.[12]

Meanwhile, B-J made a major contribution to his students outside Trumbull, in a committee room. He served, of course, on a variety of committees, including the council of masters that brought together the heads of the various colleges. But, at a time when 40 percent of the students needed work to help pay their expenses, B-J did no more important job than to chair the university's committee on bursary appointments—jobs assisting the masters, working in the libraries, researching for the faculty, and so forth. A conservative at heart, he approached the question of how to support needy students with a determination to administer the available money fairly and to exact full value for it. No portion of the bursary funds, he insisted, should go for scholarships, and students must work the full number of hours they contracted for, regardless of inconvenience.

11. Stanhope Bayne-Jones, Trumbull College: Annual Report to the President for the Year July 1, 1935 to June 30, 1936, pp. 2–3, 13, 15, 17, 20, 23, in C-42, Box 17, SBJC; Bayne-Jones to Angell, January 8, 1934, in James Rowland Angell Presidential Papers, Box 183, SML.

12. Phillips interview, 304.

The chief beneficiaries were those who were not, by background
or wealth, Yale insiders. B-J understood the big men on campus—as a
student he had been fairly big himself—but he understood the outsiders, too, for he had started at Yale as one of them. As master of
Trumbull, he was well aware that the lonely, often poor little men on
campus were the ones who most frequently participated in college
doings, because they had no social life outside; they filled the bursary
appointments, making themselves useful to himself and Nan and to the
other masters. The importance he attached to them was reflected in his
devotion to the obscure, onerous and tedious work of providing them a
livelihood on campus.[13]

B-J viewed his time at Trumbull as one of the most satisfying of
his life, and it may have been the happiest of Nan's. He learned, as he
could not in any other post, to sense the pulse of the undergraduates
for whom Yale existed in the first place. Yet hardly had he gotten well
into his task when another, much heavier one was laid atop it. In 1935
he was named dean of Yale's medical school, a post that suddenly made
him one of the most visible men in the medical profession. When control over the disposition of very large research funds followed, he also
became one of the most powerful.

That Dean Winternitz had remade Yale's medical school in the years
since 1920 no one doubted, least of all B-J: "A relatively poor school,"
he wrote, "whose abandonment was contemplated, was brought by him
and his associates into the very first group of medical institutions." Winternitz had hired distinguished faculty, had transformed a sort of technical school into a full-fledged part of the university, and had introduced the "full-time" system under which clinical professors worked for
their salaries alone, instead of teaching part-time while they practiced
medicine. He had reformed the curriculum, established a school of
nursing, found new sources of income to support the institution he had
remade, and built new structures to house it.

13. Minutes of Meetings of the Committee on the Bursary Plan, March 13, 1934, to
June 26, 1936, p. 13, in C-42, Box 17, SBJC.

For better or worse, he was a man with a vision, one that he shared in great measure with President Angell. Well aware that social disorder and poverty helped to spread disease, the two believed that medicine should contribute to the care of the whole person, as an individual and a part of society, and should work for prevention as well as cure.

A distinctive product of the Winternitz-Angell regime was the Yale Institute of Human Relations, variously described as a bold innovation and an interdepartmental stew. A research organization rather than one devoted to teaching or to patient care, the institute was originally a meeting place for psychiatrists, sociologists, and child-welfare specialists. But once take Man as the subject of study, and what could be excluded? Both medicine and law were drawn in, as investigation moved inward to the central nervous system and outward to the sources of crime and social disorder.

The institute received Winternitz' enthusiastic support. He realized that human beings are more than the sum of the parts into which the sciences, physical and social, had divided them. But B-J—and others on the faculty—saw the institute as an attempt by the dean to "take the whole university into his bailiwick and give it another name."[14]

Despite his great accomplishments, Winternitz was not a popular dean. Preventing social problems did not necessarily attract colleagues who viewed medicine as a distinct calling, primarily devoted to research and the cure of disease. For the same reason, not all were happy over the way medical studies had been lumped in with other disciplines. Winternitz' sheer fertility in new ideas was upsetting, and his autocratic ways were hard to tolerate. At the end of 1934, when the question arose whether Yale should reappoint him dean for a fourth

14. Stanhope Bayne-Jones, Report to President and Fellows of Yale University, August 31, 1936, pp. 1–2, in Yale University School of Medicine: Dean's Report, 1935–1940, in C-42, Box 17, SBJC; Phillips interview, 368. See also Arthur Viseltear, "Milton C. Winternitz and the Yale Institute of Human Relations," Yale Journal of Biology and Medicine, LVII (1984), 869; Milton C. Winternitz, "The Institute of Human Relations at Yale University," New England Journal of Medicine, CCII (January 9, 1930), 57. Also of interest is Winternitz, "A New Educational Pattern," Clinical Medicine and Surgery, XXXVIII (July, 1931), 473–75; Winternitz, "A Physician Looks at Mental Hygiene," Mental Hygiene, XVI (April, 1932), 221–32; and Yale's Plan for a Coordinated Study of Man, in Institute of Human Relations, YRG 37-V, Series 2, Box 6, SML.

five-year term, many of the senior faculty—including some recruited by Winternitz—said no.[15]

B-J was not among "Winter's" enemies. Either out of loyalty or an acute political sense, he voted to keep the old dean. Yet he sat on the faculty committee whose majority voted against Winternitz; the vote was taken in his office at Trumbull; and the committee at the same meeting voted a resolution "that Dr. Stanhope Bayne-Jones be nominated for Dean of the School of Medicine for a term of five years beginning July 1, 1935."

In a painful interview, B-J and the medical school's doyen, Harvey Cushing, delivered the news to Winternitz. Cushing presented the recommendation (now endorsed by the senior faculty) to Angell, and the president unwillingly faced up to the demotion of a man he valued and agreed with on many questions of policy. Warned that the Yale Corporation was also friendly to Winternitz' ideas, B-J gave the necessary assurances: "I have no desire to attempt to bring about any essential reversal of the broad policies now governing the development of the School." The denouement was quick. On the 12th of December, the corporation informed B-J of his appointment as dean; on the 16th a university press release announced that "Dr. Milton C. Winternitz . . . has declined to be considered for reappointment"; and on the 17th B-J gratefully accepted his new post.[16]

Behind the changeover lay emotion more than anything else—the faculty's exasperation with Winternitz and its yearning for stability, conservative management, and an end to experimentation. B-J belonged to the medical school by virtue of his status as professor of bacteriology and yet, because Trumbull absorbed most of his time, was not an active party to its inner quarrels. In more than a year at Yale he had become known to his colleagues, demonstrated his skill as a committeeman, and successfully performed an important administrative job. His professional reputation was more than ever secure, for the new edition of the *Textbook* had been issued in 1934 to a chorus of reviewers' praise.

15. Yale University General Hospital Society, *The Human Welfare Group, New Haven, Connecticut, For the Promotion of Health, Physical and Mental, Individual and Social* (New Haven, 1929), 8.

16. Recommendation on the appointment of SBJ, December 17, 1934, with accompanying memos, Angell to Bayne-Jones, January 2, 1935, Bayne-Jones to Angell, January 7, 1935, all in C-35(1), Box 16, SBJC.

In two critical ways he differed sharply from his predecessor: his personality was soothing rather than abrasive; and he was a Yale man in a university that liked to appoint its own. Both Winternitz and Angell were outsiders—brilliant ones, everybody admitted, while B-J probably was not expected to set Long Island Sound on fire. That too was in his favor. For the time being, the medical school had had quite enough of that sort of thing.

Yet B-J himself believed that one final negative element may have been decisive. He was the only member of the faculty whose appointment Winternitz would not have fought bitterly and, with support from Angell and some members of the corporation, probably with success. B-J was different. When he told "Winter" he would allow the faculty to nominate him, the old dean said, "B-J, if it's you, it's all right. If it had been somebody else, I would have fought them." B-J received the crown at least in part because Winternitz was still strong enough to deny it to anybody else in the School of Medicine.[17]

As the product of a conservative revolution, his business was to prune and clarify his predecessor's formidable legacy. He did not really have to choose between prevention and cure, or between scientific and social medicine. His duties were to improve relations with the faculty, select the best possible students from among the throngs who now applied to Yale, straighten out relationships with the university and the institute, and get secure sources of money to fund basic research into major diseases. B-J faced certain problems in satisfying both Angell, who expected him to defend his predecessor's policies, and his colleagues, who expected him to change them. But those who believe that circles cannot be squared have no business in high office.

After Winternitz, he had no reason to complain of the faculty's quality. Cushing, who had come to Yale on his retirement from Harvard, was a whole department in himself. His friend and literary executor, John F. Fulton, was a central figure in the development of

17. Phillips interview, 383. In *Treetops: A Family Memoir* (New York, 1990), 54–61, Susan Cheever (daughter of novelist John Cheever and granddaughter of Winternitz) gives a colorful version of B-J's role in her grandfather's loss of the deanship. Her account is in no sense history.

neurophysiology and neurology. Charles-Edward Amory Winslow, an eloquent and innovative prophet of social medicine, headed the department of public health. In the Institute of Human Relations, Robert M. Yerkes pioneered the study of primate behavior; his department of comparative psychobiology was a Winternitz inspiration that had worked. But to single out individuals is somewhat deceptive; Yale was strong in all major departments.[18]

The School of Medicine was a complex filling two city blocks on the east and west sides of Cedar Street. Adjacent stood the New Haven Hospital and Dispensary, a municipal treatment center like Bellevue in New York and Charity in New Orleans. Specialists from the school staffed it, and third- and fourth-year medical students studied and worked with patients on its wards. Around the hospital clustered buildings that housed bacteriology, immunology, pathology, and the clinical departments. Across the street stood the building that housed the Sterling Hall of Medicine and the Institute of Human Relations. A cramped medical library and cages of experimental animals were crowded into the Sterling, along with offices, classrooms, and laboratories. The department of psychiatry and mental hygiene belonged to the institute but also had an indefinite connection to the medical school.

In poor neighborhoods beyond the complex, eating their meals in lunchrooms, lived the medical students, some in rented rooms and some in shabby houses the university had bought or leased as impromptu dormitories. Hundreds of thousands of dollars were available for research, but little to house or feed students, many of whom, like the poorer undergraduates, lived close to the edge of penury, in "squalid quarters in the New Haven slums."[19]

Budgetary pressure affected the school as well as the students.

18. Bayne-Jones, MS Review of Fulton's *Harvey Cushing: A Biography* (Springfield, Ill., 1946), in D-1, Box 18, SBJC; Jack D. Pressman, "John F. Fulton and the Origins of Psychosurgery," *Bulletin of the History of Medicine and Allied Sciences*, LXII (Spring, 1988), 1–22; Elliot S. Valenstein, *Great and Desperate Cures: The Rise and Decline of Psychosurgery and Other Radical Treatments for Mental Illness* (New York, 1986), 78–79, 112, 147–48, 261–67.

19. Phillips interview, 407; see also Bayne-Jones, "The Yale University School of Medicine: The Educational Program for a Technical and Idealistic Profession," *The Yale Scientific Magazine* (Fall, 1936), n.p. Bayne-Jones's complaints about the poor quality of student housing and food are an annual feature of his reports as dean.

The relatively small endowment made deficits standard, and the university, in making up the shortfall from its general revenues, denied the legitimate needs of others. B-J began his term by curtailing departmental budgets, an unenviable task if only because faculties tend to view deans as nuisances whose proper business is to get them money for their pet projects, and otherwise not to interfere. In his lively, waspish diary, Fulton recorded his belief that a "rather dull and unprogressive regime, motivated largely by reactionary tendencies," was beginning.[20]

Yet B-J apparently proved himself during the first two years of his administration, despite having to serve as the "punitive agent of the depression." The legacy of mistrust between dean and faculty was embodied in a system of committees intended to restrain executive power. B-J wished to retain a single group—the Prudential Committee—which, while giving the faculty a sense of participation and limited real power, met with B-J and was subject to his influence. The willingness of the faculty to go along with this recentralization indicated growing trust and the burial of old quarrels.[21]

Other problems were more obdurate. However excellent, Yale remained a relatively small school in a small city, and relations between New Haven and the university were poor. In a time of short money, the city had to provide a variety of services for a large community in its very heart that paid no property taxes. The response of the local politicians was to refuse funds to New Haven Hospital, penalizing the sick poor who had few advocates and compelling the university to make up deficits from its own funds in order to have a teaching hospital for its medical students. Local physicians were alternately cordial to the school and resentful of the free treatment it provided to patients, many of whom (in the practitioners' opinion) could well have paid fees to men in practice.[22]

Questions of money, power, and privilege also affected admissions policy. The poverty of many students was disturbing; fully half of the

20. Diary of John F. Fulton, October 28, 1935, in Medical Historical Library, Sterling School of Medicine, Yale University.

21. Phillips interview, 402. See also Bayne-Jones, Yale University School of Medicine: Dean's Report, 1935–1940, in C-42, Box 17, SBJC; and Report, Dean to President and Fellows of Yale University, August 31, 1936, pp. 6–8, 10, 12, 21–24.

22. Phillips interview, 403–404.

applicants in 1935, if accepted, would have needed grants, scholarships, or jobs to support themselves. With funds declining, B-J steered toward a practical though harsh solution. Very brilliant students continued to be admitted and supported as necessary. But through the Prudential Committee—acting now as a committee on admissions—he restricted the number of new students who must depend upon the school for support.

In the question of minority admissions another kind of restriction came into play. Jews submitted over 40 percent of the applications received by the School of Medicine. Winternitz, a Jew bitterly resentful of his heritage, had introduced a quota system that allocated about 10 percent of each entrance class to Jews. This B-J continued without change, viewing it as generous rather than the reverse—"about three times the proportional representation of the Jewish element in the general population," he wrote in a confidential report. Other minorities won admittance but no more. A small number of women studied medicine under him, as they had under Winternitz, and B-J apparently reversed a policy of his predecessor by resuming an older Yale practice of admitting a few black students. Overall, however, getting a medical education at Yale remained incomparably easier for the qualified applicant who was prosperous, male, gentile, and white.[23]

Personal conviction and the search for funds were both reflected in B-J's modification of "full-time." Once a rallying cry of reformers in medical education, the exclusion of practicing physicians from the faculty in favor of full-time professors had proved, in practice, divisive and controversial. B-J thought the idea dubious at best, for who was to communicate to students the realities of the ordinary doctor's life if such men were shut out of teaching? In any case, Yale lacked the money to pay adequate salaries to all its clinical faculty. Cautiously, alleging that the terms of the Rockefeller grant which had originally brought full-time to Yale permitted experimentation, B-J began to allow doctors to

23. Dean's Report, August 31, 1936, especially pp. 22–24; Report for the Year 1936–37, pp. 4–5, 8, 31; Report for 1939–40, p. 20. On admission of blacks, see Nan to Peter [Olch, then deputy chief of the History of Medicine Division, NLM], May 23, 1971, Bayne-Jones Correspondence File, NLM. On Yale anti-semitism, see Oren, *Joining the Club*, especially 139–52.

receive fees from patients in the hospital and clinic who were able to pay. He secured from the university permission to transfer other fees, earned by Yale physicians who were on full salary, into a fund to provide free hospital beds for indigent cases of educational interest.

Obtaining money for research absorbed much of B-J's time and effort. Like his predecessor, he proved to be an energetic pursuer of the foundation dollar. He was well aware that New Deal taxation had made the establishment of foundations more attractive than ever to the rich, and grants earmarked for research increased yearly under his guidance. New funding heartened the department of psychiatry and mental hygiene, which in 1938 became a part of the School of Medicine. B-J took a special hand in securing money from the Yale Corporation to assist Yerkes' work, earning his passionate gratitude: "It is, I am certain, only because of your extraordinary insight, tact, sympathy, wisdom, and pains that I was able to carry on and to come back to usefulness," he wrote B-J in 1940. "No, I am not exaggerating."[24]

For one major achievement, B-J could claim only peripheral credit—the building of a new medical library at Yale. As new books jammed the shelves, B-J felt "an almost intolerable sense of a brain growing too large for its rigid case." But the decisive goad to action came from Harvey Cushing. The redoubtable surgeon wanted Yale to house his own collection, and he threatened to will his books to Johns Hopkins if it did not. Faced with the prospective loss, the corporation at last agreed to spend $600,000 for a library attached to the Hall of Medicine. The new facility not only provided medical students a working library but, through Cushing's collection, also became a center for scholarly research into medical history.[25]

B-J was far too pragmatic to either oppose or blindly endorse

24. Yerkes to Bayne-Jones, February 5, 1940, in C-37(3), Box 16, SBJC; Dean's Report, August 31, 1936, pp. 27–31; Report for 1938–39, pp. 19–20, 33, 39. See also T. W. Farnam to Bayne-Jones, February 19, 1937, in Institute of Human Relations, Series 2, Box 6, SML.

25. Phillips interview, 374; Dean's Report, 1936–37, pp. 43–44; Dean's Report, 1937–38, p. 48; Dean's Report, 1938–39, pp. 45, 46–48. The new library opened on June 15, 1941. See also Fulton's printed Christmas letters, which describe progress year by year, and his address to the Cushing Society, October 4, 1946, "On Being a Literary Executor," which gives further details. All in D-1, Box 18, SBJC.

government-insured health care. Since World War I the American Medical Association had solidified in opposition to compulsory, and even to voluntary, forms of health insurance. Shaping its public stance was an idealized image of the traditional individual medical practitioner, beholden to none but his patients and his conscience. With such an ideology B-J could feel only limited sympathy. He had never had a practice, had always worked for a salary, and had devoted his professional life to education and research. To his friend Pat O'Brien he privately expressed cautious support of federal health insurance; as dean, he confined himself to limited and concrete action.[26]

One need was real and evident in the medical school itself. A number of students were infected with tuberculosis; their work exposed them to disease, and their poor housing and diet contributed to many illnesses, especially during what B-J called the "pestilential year" of 1938 to 1939. Hence he launched a private hospitalization service plan under which each medical student contributed ten dollars and received in turn full hospital care and free medical attention from the faculty. The fund met a pressing need, and its success led B-J to urge that Yale consider a similar plan for all students. Such private health plans spread rapidly during the thirties, until the AMA leadership—pressed by members whose patients could not pay their bills and threatened by federal action—yielded. Voluntary, often doctor-controlled, plans were a mark of the time, and B-J's small contribution fitted nicely into the new orthodoxy of American medicine.[27]

Overall, however, his tenure as dean was marked by solid achievement but few new ideas. If any of the faculty had hoped for or feared a reactionary regime, they were disappointed. B-J preserved most of Winternitz' initiatives and worked with the Institute of Human Rela-

26. See Ronald L. Numbers, *Almost Persuaded: American Physicians and Compulsory Health Insurance, 1912–1920* (Baltimore, 1978); Garceau, *Political Life of the AMA*, 57, 105; James G. Burrow, *AMA: The Voice of American Medicine* (Baltimore, 1963), 184–85; Elton Raynack, *Professional Power and American Medicine: The Economics of the American Medical Association* (Cleveland, 1967), 2; Daniel F. Hirschfield, *The Lost Reform: The Campaign for Compulsory Health Insurance in the United States from 1932 to 1943* (Cambridge, Mass., 1970), 49. The contrast in outlook between professors and practitioners has been ably developed in Ludmerer, *Learning to Heal*, 129–38.

27. Dean's Report, 1938–39, pp. 31–32.

tions on common problems. He took a stand for medical humanism, supporting the contemporary movement to require a broader education and fewer scientific courses for premedical students. He kept the elective system for medical students and urged courses in the social and legal aspects of medicine, medical ethics, and the problems of practice. His primary changes were in personality and tone: he demonstrated respect for the faculty, cooled the rhetoric of social medicine, and slowed without halting the pace of innovation. Basically, he aimed to succeed, and to avoid Winternitz' fate by satisfying those who had elected him.

Subject to those limits, B-J took readily to his job, endured its pace, and loved what he called the "absurd popcorn life" it compelled the Bayne-Joneses to lead. "Nan and I," he told Pat O'Brien, "meet occasionally to exchange a few words at dinner parties at other people's houses." B-J's sense of humor did not desert him under stress, and it helped him to recognize the limits of his authority. Should a dean try to be a tsar? he asked mockingly. He felt more often like "a Tsardean . . . a poor fish that runs (in) a School and is inevitably canned after being boiled in oil."[28]

In his reports, such matters as organization and committees took less space after 1936. The faculty were getting along well; by mid-1937 the Prudential Committee was functioning as he had wanted it to. In the same year he resigned as master of Trumbull, relieving himself of a burden that he could not have carried at all during the two years past, except for Nan. With a little time now at his disposal, his old enthusiasm for research reawoke.

A subject that had interested him for several years, though he had found small opportunity to pursue it, was the use of chemicals to break down bacterial toxins. His investigations began in a small laboratory

28. Bayne-Jones to O'Brien, November 28, 1936, in A-32, Box 7, SBJC. See also Howell Cheney to Bayne-Jones, October 15, 1937, in School of Medicine: Records of the Dean, YRG 27-A-(5 to 9), Accession 1/1/61, Box 25, SML. See also Fulton Diary, February 13, 1937; Bayne-Jones, "Instruction of Students and Interns in the Legal, Social and Economic Influences Affecting Medical Practice," *AMA Bulletin* (March, 1936).

where he worked as time permitted, supervising a single assistant and a laboratory technician. Later, a Jewish refugee joined them—Alfred Cohn, formerly of the Robert Koch Institute in Berlin. Apparently Cohn's project was gotten up to afford him employment, for he researched the gonococcus, a subject in which he was an expert but B-J had only passing interest. B-J liked and admired him and actively pursued money to support his work from the national committees—Jewish groups, the American Friends Service Committee, and the Federal Council of Churches of Christ—that provided aid to refugees. He valued his little laboratory, the refuge it provided him, and the contact with like-minded people.[29]

While enjoying his own work, he maintained a generous interest in that of his colleagues. Deficient in jealousy, he liked to see the men and women around him accomplishing greater things than he could hope to. Winternitz, though bitter, resumed his earlier specialty and did prizewinning work in pathology. An interdepartmental group studied the electrodynamics of living systems. Faculty members did important research on polio—primarily on the multiplicity of viral strains and the means of transmission. Cushing's registry of different types of brain tumors grew steadily. Fulton's laboratory remained a center of research into the nervous system; he cofounded the *Journal of Neurophysiology* and in 1938 published his masterpiece, *The Physiology of the Nervous System.*[30]

Studies of cancer, an interest with several Yale scientists, continued under a patchwork of grants and bequests. An interdepartmental group set up by Winternitz, the Atypical Growth Study Unit, brought together those who were interested in tumors. B-J gave cancer no par-

29. Dean's Report, 1936–37, p. 2. See also Bayne-Jones, Report of S. Bayne-Jones' Division of the Department of Bacteriology, June 14, 1935, and Report of Bacteriology (B–J), July 1, 1940–June 30, 1941, both in C-47, Box 17, SBJC; and his yearly note on the same subject in the Dean's Reports. On Bayne-Jones's efforts to support Cohn, see Cecilia Raznovsky to Bayne-Jones, March 26, 1936, and Bayne-Jones to George Baehr, July 2, 1935, both in School of Medicine, Records of the Dean, Box 27, SML. Raznovsky represented the National Coordinating Committee for Aid to Refugees and Emigrants Coming from Germany, and Baehr represented the Emergency Committee in Aid of Displaced Foreign Physicians.

30. Dean's Report, 1936–37, pp. 55, 71, 76, and 1937–38, pp. 67, 100; John F. Fulton, *The Physiology of the Nervous System* (London, 1938); Saul Benison, *Tom Rivers: Reflections on a Life in Medicine and Science* (Cambridge, Mass., 1967), 262–70.

ticular thought—it was simply one of many research endeavors that he tried to support—until January 5, 1937. On that day a telephone call brought the first hint that a multimillionaire was interested in the disease and that an enormous gift for Yale might be at hand.

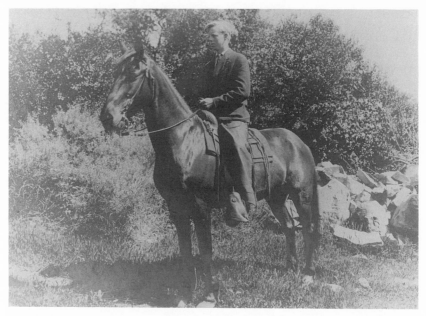

Stanhope Bayne-Jones on horseback at Thacher School in California, *ca.* 1906
Courtesy National Library of Medicine

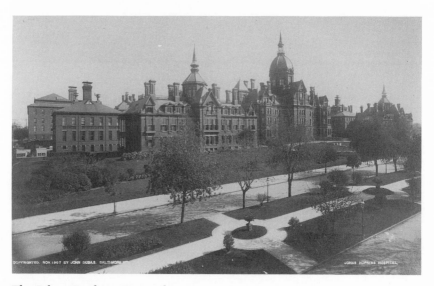

The Johns Hopkins Hospital in 1907
Photograph by John Dubas. Courtesy National Library of Medicine

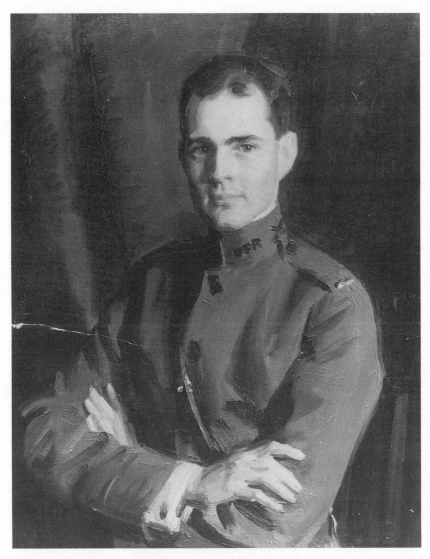

Howard Vincent "Pat" O'Brien in World War I uniform
Courtesy National Library of Medicine

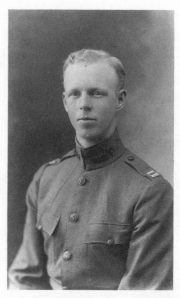

Bayne-Jones as a captain in the United States Army Medical Corps, *ca.* 1917
Courtesy National Library of Medicine

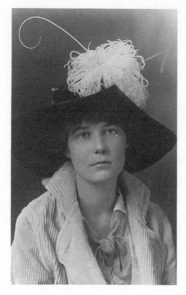

Nan Smith Bayne-Jones as a young woman, 1921
Courtesy National Library of Medicine

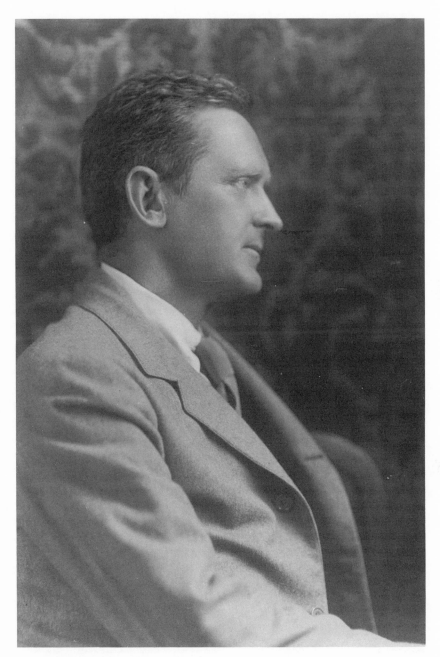

Hans Zinsser
Courtesy National Library of Medicine

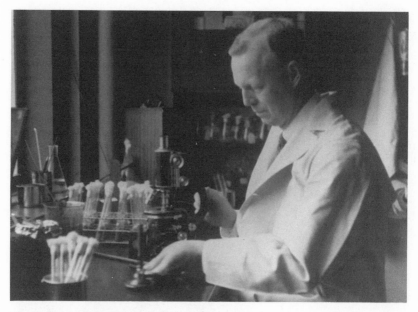

Bayne-Jones in his laboratory at Yale, *ca.* 1938
Courtesy National Library of Medicine

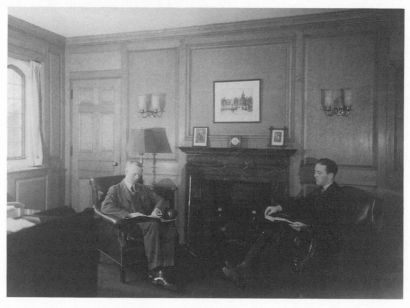

Bayne-Jones in his study at Trumbull College, where he was master
Courtesy National Library of Medicine

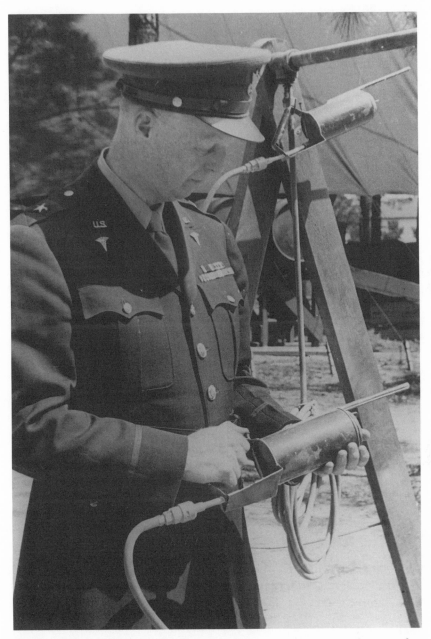

Bayne-Jones inspects a dust gun—his favorite weapon—used to combat typhus during World War II

Courtesy National Library of Medicine

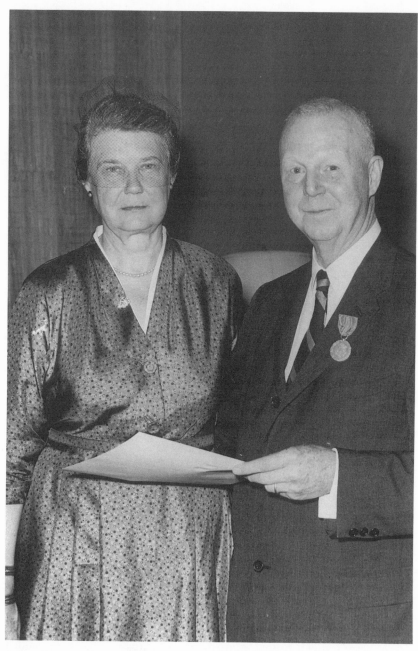

Bayne-Jones and Nan at his retirement from the army, 1956
Courtesy National Library of Medicine

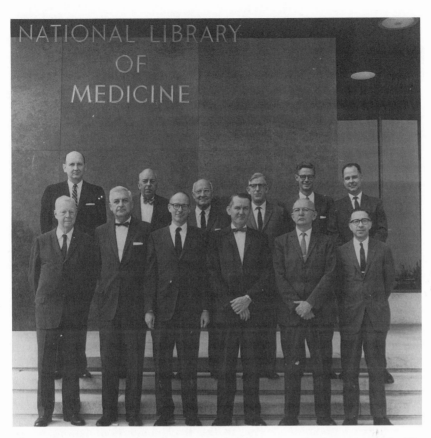

The Surgeon General's Advisory Committee on Smoking and Health.
Bayne-Jones is on the front row, far left
Courtesy National Library of Medicine

SEVEN

Power and Loss

A man identifying himself as Dr. John S. Dye said that he wished to discuss the possibility of a gift to Yale research. Dye turned out to be a surgeon, practicing in Waterbury. He was "quite mysterious." He would identify the prospective donor only as a Yale graduate living in Connecticut. They chatted, and Dye went away.[1]

There for almost a week the matter rested. Then Dye called to say that he had arranged a meeting in New York with the still nameless philanthropist. The morning of January 13 found B-J and Dye on a train to the city, where they were greeted in a Park Avenue apartment by a somewhat deaf old man named Starling W. Childs. Childs and B-J settled into a window alcove for a private talk.

B-J learned that Childs's medical interests were confined to diseases that had touched him directly—hearing loss, because of his own disability; poliomyelitis, because one of his sons had been crippled in the 1916 epidemic; and cancer, because his wife, the former Julia Coffin, had died of the disease. Determined to use his fortune to fight one or more of these ills, Childs had weighed various alternatives—setting up his own foundation, giving to the Rockefeller Foundation, or bestowing funds on a medical school. B-J adopted a tone of helpful objectivity, pointing out advantages and disadvantages to each. Then, zeroing in, he gave a lengthy account of Yale's work in the field of cancer, underlining the efforts of Winternitz' Atypical Growth Study Unit. In conclusion, he candidly said that he hoped Childs would give the money to Yale.

On this subject Childs already had some clear ideas. The possible donation would be in the form of securities; the university would be the trustee, but Childs intended to control the management of the funds through a board of managers of his own appointing. B-J, pointing

1. Bayne-Jones, Memorandum for Cancer Research Fund, n.d., in D-17(5), Box 19, SBJC; see also Harvey to Bayne-Jones, January 4, 1937, *ibid.* This account from primary sources differs in detail from Bayne-Jones's recollections in Phillips interview, 445–46.

out that he could not commit Yale, asked Childs to a luncheon *à trois* with himself and the university treasurer. As to what all this might lead to, B-J noted in his memorandum of the meeting that "Dr. Dye seems to think it will be a million or more."[2]

When he learned the true extent of Childs' fortune, B-J's hopes became stronger. Apparently, the philanthropist's dead wife was the source of most of the wealth, through her family's holdings in General Electric. In any case, Childs was a very rich man, and his "summer place" at Norfolk was an estate. B-J became more and more excited as the day set for the luncheon—January 18—approached. Childs arrived in New Haven with a general plan for the donation in hand. In essence, the fund was to be administered by a director, a board of trustees, and a scientific advisory board. The trustees would manage the investments, while the advisory board selected the projects and the director coordinated the whole. Though Childs intended to see Yale become a major center of research, he wished support to be given also to worthy projects elsewhere. The causes of cancer, rather than the cure, were to be sought first, and investigations into polio were also to receive aid. He had tentatively named the endeavor the Childs Fund for Medical Research.[3]

B-J and the university were still digesting this proposal when a new bombshell arrived from Park Avenue. Childs's sister-in-law, Alice Coffin—a shy spinster who occupied another apartment in his building—wished to join the fight against cancer. "She is very much interested," he wrote, "and if 'things can be arranged' wants to contribute to the 'Jane Coffin Childs Fund for Medical Research' as we now propose to call it. If things work out as they are now headed, I can see that 5 millions may easily be the *minimum* and it may reach to higher figures." B-J may well have felt that he was living in a dream.[4]

Meetings followed in which the organization took form. At Childs's own insistence, B-J emerged as an important figure, prospectively the

2. Bayne-Jones, Memorandum For Cancer Research Fund, in D-17(5), Box 19, SBJC.
3. Bayne-Jones to Starling W. Childs, January 18, 1937, Edward C. Childs to Bayne-Jones, January 19, 1937, both *ibid*. See also Phillips interview, 447.
4. Childs to Bayne-Jones, n.d., Bayne-Jones to Childs, February 1, 1937, both in D-17(5), Box 19, SBJC.

head of the scientific advisory board. The organization received its final name: The Jane Coffin Childs Memorial Fund for Medical Research. With the basics settled, a lengthy round of gentlemanly negotiation followed, in a succession of luncheons, a flurry of letters, and a salvo of compliments. The draft proposal was reviewed again and again; changes were entered and in some cases changed back. As the work proceeded, B-J emerged as the go-between, a matchmaker nailing down the last details of a marriage both sides now felt committed to.

The result was a plan that met the agendas, open or hidden, of the philanthropist, of Yale, and of B-J himself. All verbiage aside, the treasurer of the board of managers was to handle the money, and B-J's advisory board was to decide how to spend it. For B-J, who was bored by money but relished power, the setup could not have been better.[5]

By mid-May, B-J had his list of nominees ready. In addition to himself, he favored Rudolph J. Anderson, Yale's premier professor of organic chemistry and biochemistry, then at work on substances that would soon be called carcinogens; Ross G. Harrison, Sterling Professor of Biology, whom B-J thought "the most distinguished scientist on the Yale faculty at this time," with a record of work on tissue cultures; Peyton Rous of the Rockefeller Institute for Medical Research, famed for his discovery that a virus could cause some cancers in birds; and Milton C. Winternitz, for his incomparable connections, talent, and energy. Childs accepted all without question. At the end of the month came one last important change. The Childs family decided to omit poliomyelitis from the targets of the fund. If the fight against cancer was won, the managers could, upon the recommendation of the scientific advisers, attack other diseases as they chose.[6]

Throughout these negotiations, B-J showed his skills to great advantage. No doubt the talent in Yale's medical school was the key to success; Childs's emotional tie to the university of which he was an alumnus played a part; but B-J's role was a crucial one. When his op-

5. Flexner to Bayne-Jones, May 7, 1937, in D-17(6), Box 19, SBJC.
6. Bayne-Jones to Childs, May 11, 1937, Bayne-Jones, Memorandum, May 31, 1937 (Child's Fund), both in D-17(8), Box 19, SBJC. See also True Copy of Prudential Committee Meeting [minutes], June 12, 1937, in D-17(9), Box 19, SBJC. Childs's decision to concentrate against cancer may have reflected the influence of Alice Coffin.

portunity came, he had the wit, the position, and the expert knowledge to seize upon it. Within a year, the Childs benefaction would supply almost one-third of Yale's new research funds.[7]

All was now complete save the final wordsmithing. By the end of the first week of June the lawyers had drafted the deed of gift. On the 12th, Yale's Prudential Committee recommended acceptance of the benefaction, and on the 21st the corporation agreed. President Angell, as one of his last acts before his retirement, announced to the Alumni Luncheon "the greatest gift yet made to Yale for the benefit of our work in the field of scientific research."[8]

The importance of the benefaction was extraordinary in the context of the time. Launched with an initial endowment of about $4 million, the fund was increased by later gifts and bequests to $10 million, "by far the largest single gift in the history of cancer philanthropy." At the time, only about two dozen funds in the United States were promoting cancer research, and their aggregate resources did not exceed $5 million. It was also true that the creation of the new fund came almost literally at the last moment that a private gift could have so marked an impact. In August, 1937, the federal government's modest commitment to fight cancer—averaging about $95,000 a year from 1930 to 1937—increased sharply with the creation of the National Cancer Institute in Bethesda, Maryland.[9]

The increase in public and private funding for research signaled a new attitude toward cancer. Like tuberculosis, venereal disease, and mental illness, cancer had long been stigmatized as an ailment too distressing and repugnant even to discuss. It was thought incurable, an act of God. Medical researchers avoided cancer for other reasons. Investigators of cancer had no ready-made key to help them unravel its mys-

7. *The Jane Coffin Childs Memorial Fund for Medical Research: The Deed of Gift, By-Laws, and other Official Documents* (New Haven, 1938), 23–24. The Dean's Report for 1937–38, p. 64, shows that the Childs Fund contributed $54,500 of $171,181.40 in new grants.

8. Dean's Report for 1936–37, p. 35, in C-42, Box 17, SBJC.

9. Patterson, *Dread Disease*, 117.

tery. After some advances during the Progressive Era, false reports of medical breakthroughs helped to make the interwar years a time of declining support and professional interest. With success unlikely and money hard to come by, many able people thought research in the field an excellent way to bury a career. (*Fortune* magazine reported in 1937 that the average cancer investigator was lucky to receive a carpenter's wages.)

Yet light had begun to appear in what the magazine called "The Great Darkness." Medical success in preventing and curing infectious disease, combined with improved nutrition and progress in public health, had created a population in which increasing numbers of people reached middle age. Life expectancy at birth increased rapidly, but at fifty it remained about the same, summoning researchers to consider the diseases characteristic of later life—cancer and hypertension among them. In 1924 recorded deaths from cancer for the first time surpassed those from tuberculosis. Ten years later the Metropolitan Life Insurance Company estimated that cancer caused about 10 percent of all deaths in the United States (134,428 out of 1,396,903) and had become the second-ranking cause of mortality after heart and vascular ailments. By the end of the 1930s, 150,000 Americans died every year from cancer, more than 1 for every 1,000 of the population. Though the nation contributed little as yet to cancer research, it spent great sums on treatment.

Hope of an ultimate cure remained no more than that. Since the time of Hippocrates, no new principle of treatment had been devised; either the cancer must be cut out or the cancerous tissue destroyed. Although aseptic surgery had replaced earlier butchery, and X rays and radium had replaced caustics, the basic approaches remained the same. Prevention was the favorite reliance, but difficult to put into practice. Doctors emphasized the importance of early detection, yet lacked instruments and techniques to discover tumors deep in the body.

By 1937, however, advances in several fields promised new understanding of how cancers were caused. The fact was well understood that the malignant tumor represented the uncontrolled multiplication of cells. Candidates for the triggering mechanism now included viruses, radiation, and carcinogenic chemicals. The study of hormones seemed to promise new clues. Experts acknowledged the existence of a hereditary predisposition to certain cancers. Considerable progress had been made in differentiating the many kinds of cancers, each with its own characteristic patterns of growth and lethality. More vigorous leadership in the American Society for the Control of Cancer matched a more receptive attitude toward government assistance under the New Deal. As funding increased, the mystery of the disease, instead of repelling, began to attract investigators. For many reasons, an American crusade began to gather against the most baffling of ills, and B-J was one of its leaders.[10]

At the age of forty-eight, B-J could be pretty sure now that he had found his métier. After all, practical things were what he did best. He was more man of the world than scientist, more doer than thinker, more Bayne than Jones. Now he stood where he had wanted to be, near the summit of American medicine. He was a powerful man, and henceforth acted and thought like one. He hoped to gain the presidency of Yale when Angell retired, and he received serious consideration before the corporation settled upon Charles Seymour, the university provost, who was credited with originating the plan for residential colleges. This disappointment may not have been a great one to B-J, for it remains unclear how seriously he had viewed his own candidacy.[11]

Yet it introduced a time of personal and professional loss that contrasted strangely with his apparently overwhelming success. One of B-J's few intimates among the vast throng of his professional acquaintances was his coauthor, Hans Zinsser. Much of their relationship centered on the textbook. But common interests and contrasting personali-

10. "Cancer: The Great Darkness," *Fortune*, XV (March, 1937), 112–13, 162–79; Patterson, *Dread Disease*, 27–28, 32, 81, 93–102. Cancer is treated in the present work as a single disease, in deference to Lewis Thomas' opinion that "all forms of cancer, in whatever organisms and of whatever types, are a single disease, caused by a central controlling mechanism gone wrong" (Lewis Thomas, *The Youngest Science: Notes of a Medicine-Watcher* [New York, 1983], 202).

11. Carter Glass to Bayne-Jones, March 8, 1937, in E-1(G), Box 22, SBJC. Pat O'Brien consoled Bayne-Jones for missing the post, saying he would be happier with the "cancer bequest" than "the presidential baton" (O'Brien to Bayne-Jones, July 8, 1937, in A-32, Box 7, SBJC). See also Fulton Diary, February 13, 1937.

ties—the sweet and salt flavors of a friendship—bound them more closely than shared work and profits. Nothing could dim Zinsser's enthusiasm and goodwill. "B-J is going to be the steady & kindly balance wheel of medical educational development in the next ten or fifteen years," he told Nan, "& people will turn to him more & more for advice & guidance. See if they don't!" And to B-J he predicted, "I expect you to develop the sort of place in your generation that Popsy Welch did in the last one."

For his own part, B-J made sure that the relationship did not die out. Squeezing in visits to Harvard as best he could, he continued to seek Zinsser out for advice, for the joys of drinking and argument, and for the somatic delight that a cool nature feels in the presence of a warm one. As he once told his friend, "a visit with you is good for the soul." [12]

Increasingly Zinsser's work centered on typhus. He and the group he headed at Harvard played essential roles in a complex, worldwide drama of discovery. Scientists gradually revealed the relationships between the rickettsial diseases—including epidemic typhus, murine typhus, trench fever, the Rocky Mountain spotted fever of America, and the *tsutsugamushi* disease of Asia—and the array of lice, fleas, ticks, and chiggers that spread them. Zinsser developed an almost brotherly feeling for lice, the small creatures that, he believed, had originally caught typhus from humankind and not the other way about. In 1935 he published *Rats, Lice and History*, a book that explored the lore of typhus and speculated on how disease had influenced humankind across the ages. A bestseller, the book showed clearly the contrast between himself and B-J: *Man and Microbes*, clear and objective, had dropped quickly from sight; *Rats, Lice and History*, fairly throbbing with the personality, crotchets, wit, and scholarship of Hans Zinsser, remains a standard more than half a century later.

About the dangers of his quest, Zinsser said little. Yet the organism that causes epidemic typhus, *Rickettsia prowazeki*, killed the two investigators for whom it was named, the American Howard Taylor Ricketts and the Austrian Stanislaus J. M. Von Prowazek. Zinsser himself caught typhus during his studies and came close to death. By the

---

12. Zinsser to Nan, n.d. [1935], Zinsser to Bayne-Jones, October 8, 1935, both in C-7(10), Box 14, SBJC. Bayne-Jones to Zinsser, November 11, 1937, in C-8(2), Box 14, *ibid.*

mid-thirties much labor and risk had narrowed the problem of making
a practical vaccine to the question of how to grow great numbers of
rickettsiae, which, like viruses, are obligate parasites unable to exist
apart from living cells. Convinced that a method he had developed
worked, Zinsser visited China in 1938 to get production started where
the disease was most destructive. He planned to carry his mission to
Europe afterward. "It will be a great thing," B-J wrote him, "if you can
establish your typhus work over there [in China] promptly and then
return to finish the job in Europe this year also." But Zinsser did not
see Europe again.[13]

He returned from Asia, he later said, "badly damaged." On the
steamer, homeward bound, he noticed that a British general his own
age outlasted him at deck tennis. The sun burned him yellow instead of
brown. Before the ship docked he had made a tentative diagnosis on
himself. In Boston he went to his personal physician, who in due time
confirmed it. Then, Zinsser later recalled, the two stood at the window
of the doctor's office, looking out on Charles River Basin. It was early
afternoon of a rare day in June, and little white sails raced along the
Cambridge shore. People strolled or sat on benches in the sunlight, and
the voices of children at play came through the open window.

In time, when he had come to the best terms he could with the
verdict, Zinsser wrote about the heightening of experience that accompanied the realization that his days were numbered, the slowing and
enriching of passing moments, the deep autumnal tones that gave accent to sights, sounds, and memories. But his letters to B-J showed that
acceptance came hard and was never complete.[14]

B-J's first intimation of trouble came shortly after the diagnosis.
Zinsser wrote him that "for the first time in my life I do *not* feel physi-
cally fit. I want to see you as soon as possible." B-J invited him to New
Haven. But a few days later he received another letter. Again Zinsser

13. For an attempt to unravel Zinsser's contributions to typhus research, see Peter K.
Olitsky, "Hans Zinsser and His Studies on Typhus Fever," *Journal of the American Medical
Association*, CXVI (March 8, 1941), 907–12. See also Bayne-Jones to Zinsser, February 18,
1938, in C-8(2), Box 14, SBJC. A functional typhus vaccine already existed but could only be
made in small quantities.

14. Zinsser, *As I Remember Him*, 437. The book is Zinsser's autobiography but takes
the form of a third-person memoir of the author's own Romantic Self.

did not name his illness, but the contents were alarming. He wrote of himself in the past tense, clearly a man who was trying to sort out the meaning of his life. Above all, he said, he was grateful for the work that he had been allowed to do. His son had pleased him by deciding to follow him into medicine. "Is there any imaginable activity—for intelligent and courageous people that can equal it?"[15]

B-J was anxious to see him, but instead had to fly to New Orleans. It was rather a sad homecoming, for Tante E had died at last, after a distressing final illness that apparently had brought on the disintegration of her excellent mind, and Bayne and Alma were selling the old house where she had reigned so long over the clan. Back in New England, however, B-J made a hasty trip to Boston. An emotional meeting followed that left Zinsser somewhat formal in the aftermath. "There are times," he wrote, "when one appreciates more than one can express the spontaneous friendship shown by people of whom one has long been fond." B-J, usually the more reserved of the two, said simply, "Thank you for the afternoon and early evening in Boston last week. I shall never forget it."[16]

Patients with leukemia often take a long time to die. The two men continued to revise the textbook, making ready for the eighth edition. Zinsser at first was able to do all his usual work and what he described as "some extra writing" as well—probably his autobiography. He tried to make postmortem arrangements, asking B-J's "transferred friendship" for his son and disclaiming any need to pay textbook royalties to his family, once the last edition he had actually worked on was superseded. When Zinsser hit slumps, he scrawled hasty letters about his illness, while forbidding B-J to mention it in return. "I'm letting out a bit of discouraged gray weather mood on your affectionate heart."[17]

Possibly at B-J's insistence (though he denied it) Yale decided to award Zinsser an honorary degree for his work on typhus. On June 21,

15. Zinsser to Bayne-Jones, June 24 and 27, 1938, in C-8(2), Box 14, SBJC.

16. Zinsser to Bayne-Jones, August 1, 1938, Bayne-Jones to Zinsser, August 5, 1938, both in C-8(2), Box 14, SBJC. Nan wrote that Bayne-Jones was "a little depressed about it going out of the family," but congratulated Alma on leaving a house whose "unpleasant memories must outnumber the happy ones" (Nan to Alma, June 28, 1938, in Bayne-Jones File, AMC).

17. Zinsser to Bayne-Jones, February 24, 1939, in C-8(3), Box 14, SBJC.

1939, Zinsser and his wife, Ruth, came to the ceremony. The award took place at commencement, amid measured academic ritual. The day was warm and bright. Zinsser rose when the Public Orator spoke his name, stepped forward facing the speaker until the introduction was over, then walked to the center of the platform to receive his diploma from Charles Seymour, Yale's new president.

Among his fellow honorees was one who had lately occupied a more visible stage. Former president Edvard Beneš of recently dismembered Czechoslovakia arrived with a gaggle of detectives to guard him from assassination. Clearly the hero of the occasion, Beneš received a standing ovation; later, at the alumni luncheon, he said, "This would seem to be the age of midnight in many parts of Europe today."[18]

Back in Boston, working on his book, Zinsser brooded about the state of science and the world. Neither seemed to be working well. Science was out of hand, and the technology it had set loose seemed self-serving and uncontrollable. In Germany the Nazis were destroying or perverting the scientific tradition Zinsser had been raised in, and many people he knew "now (& rightly) hate everything German."

Yet a late sonnet Zinsser wrote to his wife declared, "Now is death merciful." And so it proved. In early 1940 he announced his method for making typhus vaccine, reaping well-earned praise for his fifteen years of work on the problem; he did not live long enough to see his method superseded by a better one. He finished his autobiography, and the Book-of-the-Month Club took it, assuring a wide sale and a larger estate for his family. In September, Zinsser entered New York's Memorial Hospital for the Treatment of Cancer and Allied Diseases, knowing that he would not leave it alive. B-J, though he directed the expenditure of millions in the fight against cancer, was as powerless as anyone else to aid him. Zinsser died at 4:30 on the morning of September 4.[19]

To B-J, Zinsser's finest work had been himself. Many who knew Zinsser thought of him not in the category of research scientists but in the company of the great clinicians or of the poets. B-J knew other sides

18. Unsigned letter of instruction to Zinsser, May 15, 1939, *ibid.*; New York *Times*, June 22, 1939; New Haven *Evening Register*, June 21, 1939.

19. Richard P. Strong, "Hans Zinsser: Bacteriologist, Teacher, Philosopher, Author, Poet, Soldier," *Science*, XCII (September 27, 1940), 276–79.

of him, including the alternate explosions of enthusiasm and rage that had made Zinsser so entrancing a companion. The ill-informed, said B-J, thought Zinsser "gently poetic," but those who knew him better found his mind incisive, keenly critical, "sometimes in a turmoil of violent opinion and expression."

Still others saw in his death the passing of an older and better Germany that had been the instructor rather than the would-be master of the Western world. In an editorial entitled "As We Remember Him," the New York *Times* recalled that Zinsser "was a man molded in the Teutonic culture whose interests were universal, whose pity was in acts rather than words, who loved wine and gayety and women's smiles, who did not aspire to power but to understanding. There are such men in Germany still, let us not doubt; there are such German souls waiting to be born; out of them can still come a Germany that will be humane and splendid."[20] That was true and moving, but for B-J the matter was simpler. Fate is a miser, and he would not have such a friend again.

Professional loss accompanied the personal. B-J had resigned his job at Trumbull to be dean of the medical school and director of the Childs fund. Then, in 1940, a sharp difference with Yale led him to refuse renomination to the deanship as well.

The event was sudden and painful. Freed from the burden of Trumbull, he was by 1939 at ease with the task of running the medical school, whose board of permanent officers unanimously endorsed him for a new five-year term. In December, President Seymour told B-J that he intended to recommend his reappointment. "I cannot remember," wrote Seymour, "any five years of a Dean's administration here more successful than yours." But B-J hedged, saying that he must reserve his decision until he and Seymour could discuss the attitude of the Yale Corporation toward a pet project, the Institute of Nutrition. His letter was uncharacteristic, for it implied a confrontation; B-J, usually so supple, intended to make a stand on an issue of substance.[21]

20. Bayne-Jones, MS article, "Hans Zinsser," 6, for *The Dictionary of American Biography*, in C-21, Box 14, SBJC; New York *Times*, September 5, 1940.
21. Seymour to Bayne-Jones, December 7, 1939, and Bayne-Jones to Seymour, December 10, 1939, both in C-37(1), Box 16, SBJC.

Most of what he had done to date as dean represented modifications or extensions of the Winternitz legacy. This project was his own. During the 1930s, food companies had begun to show interest in medical research, especially on vitamins. In November, 1938, Charles Wesley Dunn, a Canadian-born New York lawyer who had long served the industry, proposed an institute of nutrition to the Associated Grocery Manufacturers of America, meeting at the Waldorf-Astoria. An enthusiast for the interests he represented, Dunn later explained his reasoning: the science of nutrition was "a basic part of preventive medicine," and yet there was "no central and coordinating instrument for the due development of this science." Consulting the president of General Foods, Dunn found him willing to join other food manufacturers to sponsor and support an institute to be set up in affiliation with "one of our great universities."

Fresh from his triumph with the Childs fund, B-J hoped to capture the institute. Perhaps he was unaware that many members of the Yale Corporation would view funding by commercial institutions as quite different from the gift of a philanthropist. B-J contacted Dunn and, with the aid of the Yale treasurer, gradually worked out a scheme by which the industry was to fund a professorship of nutrition at Yale, sponsor research, and help to educate young people in the field. From the beginning, control was a problem; when B-J sought "almost complete control" of the institute for the university, Dunn withdrew, and the talks lapsed for a time. B-J made concessions, and by the spring of 1939 things were moving again, despite murmurs of opposition from within Yale. Many people were intrigued by what the president of the Carnegie Corporation called "a constructive collaboration between business and the universities, for public benefit." Vannevar Bush expressed interest; the opportunity seemed good to bring major new funds into an important area of basic research.[22]

For a time all seemed to go well. President Seymour and the Yale Prudential Committee endorsed the negotiations. B-J hoped for contri-

22. Bayne-Jones to Thomas D. Thacher [a lawyer and member of the Yale Corporation], January 22, 1940, Dunn to D. E. Montgomery, Consumer Counsel, Agricultural Adjustment Administration, June 9, 1939, both in School of Medicine, Records of the Dean, YRG 27-A-(5 to 9), Accession 1/1/61, Box 69, SML.

butions from Julius Fleischmann, Standard Brands, and the National Biscuit Company, and invitations to contribute went out to Borden, Heinz, Campbell, National Dairy, Beech-Nut, General Mills, and others. An architect drew up preliminary plans for a building to house the institute, and Yale began to look for a donor. If B-J was straying down the garden path, Dunn was no less caught up in the project he had fathered, which he saw as a source both of basic and applied research, and as a means of educating the public in sound nutrition.

But the Yale Corporation's committee on the Institute of Nutrition, led by future Secretary of State Dean G. Acheson, had other ideas. The members objected to the method of funding—the manufacturers wanted to finance by annual, rather than long-term, grants—and to the influence the manufacturers would exert on the institute through the members they would appoint to its board of governors. Some Yale representatives envisioned the institute becoming a new means of corporate advertisement (Yale endorses Campbell soups) and demanded complete control of the institute for the university. Faced with opposition, Seymour withdrew his support. This *volte-face* typified a less than admirable side of Yale's new president. A man of find mind, suave manner, and considerable warmth, Seymour liked to evade firm commitments. The committee's opposition and his reversal boded ill for the project. By spring, Dunn had abandoned Yale and was negotiating with Arthur Compton of the Massachusetts Institute of Technology.[23]

B-J had invested considerable effort, time, prestige, and ego in the project. Yale's determination to avoid the soiling touch of commerce deprived him not only of another coup but of the most original initiative of his tenure as dean—a chance to make a fundamental contribution to preventive medicine through an imaginative collaboration between industry and academe. He protested, then refused to serve as Yale's agent in presenting terms he knew would be rejected. Within the month his decision on the deanship was due. After talking to Seymour, he announced that he would not be a candidate.

The president was shocked; the medical school's board of perma-

23. Kelley, *Yale: A History*, 394; Phillips interview, 410–15, 495; Bayne-Jones to Seymour, December 10, 1939, in School of Medicine, Records of the Dean, Box 137, SML. See also material in C-37(1), Box 16, SBJC.

nent officers asked B-J to reconsider. His colleagues reacted in a variety of ways. Some commiserated with him; others, believing B-J's protestations about his love of research, congratulated him on ridding himself of a burden. Acheson was not deceived. In a letter mingling apologies with thanks to B-J for kindness to his son, then a freshman at Yale, Acheson expressed the hope that "friendship survives even a judgment of error."

But B-J's deanship did not. He had surrendered a post he thoroughly liked in a mood of indignation and injured pride. He tried to explain his motives to his old roommate Pat O'Brien, arguing that he had been betrayed. Pat, however, found his explanation less than clear. "I still puzzle at your story," he wrote. "There is still something about it that baffles me." Though B-J never sought to withdraw his abrupt decision, he regretted its consequences: "I really was sorry to go," he admitted, many years later.[24]

Publicly, B-J gave the excuse that he wished to devote full time to the Childs fund, to his research in the field of bacteriology, and to a university fund-raising committee for medicine and public health. None of the claims had much merit. The Childs fund work was heavy but intermittent. B-J had, if anything, a lower estimate of his modest abilities in the laboratory than the facts warranted. The fund-raising committee accomplished little. As B-J remarked ruefully, the financing of the medical school was, after all, the business of the new dean, Francis G. Blake. The chief result of the fund-raising effort was to give B-J his most jaw-breaking title ever: Chairman of the Executive Committee of the Division of Medicine and Public Health of the President's Committee on University Development—academic bureaucracy in a nutshell.[25]

Losing the deanship did not, of course, leave him idle. The habit

24. Dean Acheson to Nan, December 14, 1939, in School of Medicine, Records of the Dean, C-39(4), Box 137, SML; O'Brien to Bayne-Jones, November 7, 1940, in C-39(4), Box 16, SBJC; and Phillips interview, 502. See also Bayne-Jones to O'Brien, November 27, 1940, in C-39(4), Box 16, SBJC.

25. Bayne-Jones to Seymour, in C-39(4), Box 16, SBJC. The official cover story is given in *Yale News*, February 16, 1940.

of juggling a whole kitchen cabinet of assorted duties was by now firm upon him. He was still professor of bacteriology. In 1939 he became a member of the board of directors of the Josiah Macy, Jr., Foundation; Zinsser inveigled him into a place on the advisory medical board of the Leonard Wood Foundation for the Eradication of Leprosy; in 1940 and 1941 he served as president of the American Association of Pathologists and Bacteriologists; from 1939 to 1941 he was a member of the board of scientific advisers of the International Health Division of the Rockefeller Foundation. His line to Washington remained open through membership on two committees of the National Research Council. All were posts of honor, involved a certain amount of work, extended his acquaintanceship, and served to take him beyond Yale to the boardrooms where decisions on national medical policy were made.

Above all, the work of the Childs fund continued heavy. The scientific advisers worked out procedures for selecting worthy projects and launched a new journal, *Cancer Research*, which B-J undertook to edit. By 1940, work funded at Yale and elsewhere was bringing about thirty technical publications a year on various aspects of the disease. But his chief work was to wrestle with questions of basic policy. Finding the proper niche for the fund was by no means simple, for the cancer-research field was changing rapidly. Increased funding at the National Cancer Institute (NCI) and around the country typified the time.

B-J was intimately involved with the early years of the NCI. He hoped it might become a central authority, coordinating the efforts of others and so preventing duplication of effort among the increasing numbers of private programs. With some central direction, each foundation might pursue an integrated program in its own area of competence, while it cooperated with all the others.

In practice, both parts of this program proved hard to achieve. Each foundation was subject to its own vested interests, to the hopes and ambitions of its staff, to honest differences of opinion as to what field of research was most promising, and to the conflicts of personalities. To do his part in seeking consensus, B-J undertook to consult with other directors, exchanging visits and inviting them to attend meetings of the Childs fund's board of scientific advisers. Some of this was genuine statesmanship, but some showed a canny medical politician at work. Much of B-J's diplomacy was intended to forestall the danger that other funds might withdraw support from Yale research. B-J intended, as his benefactor did, to keep the bulk of the Childs fund grants in New Haven; to do so while persuading outsiders that Yale still needed and deserved their money as well was no easy task. Hence the board made grants to Washington University in Saint Louis and to Johns Hopkins at least partly to show that the fund was a national and not a local philanthropy.[26]

Yet B-J's dedication to the cancer fight, beginning as a professional commitment, grew more personal and intense as the disease struck down close friends and relatives. In pursuit of integrated and cooperative effort, B-J attended some Washington meetings of the National Advisory Cancer Council, which had been set up to provide scientific direction to the NCI. He found the high-powered group willing to act as an information clearinghouse. NCI's own role was becoming clearer; it would support its own research but also make grants in aid elsewhere.[27]

But the Childs fund advisers still sought a function to call their own. "A foundation in search of a program," said B-J, "is a common wandering sort of a creature." Should they recommend many small grants, or back only one line of research—on viruses, for example, or on carcinogenic substances? Discussions of policy always led back to individuals and to individual achievements. "The programs have turned out to be mere articulated dry bones," said Rous, and B-J agreed. "The essential vital elements are the investigators," he emphasized, and discovery was like the wind that "bloweth where it listeth."

Yet they felt uncomfortable with a policy of pure opportunism. By early 1938 the advisers had decided to back a number of carefully se-

26. Report of November 8, 1937, pp. 1–5, 8–9, in The Jane Coffin Childs Fund for Medical Research: Reports of the Director, Board of Scientific Advisers, to the Board of Managers for the Period July 1, 1937 to May 14, 1940, in D-18, Box 19, SBJC. The makeup of the board of scientific advisers tended to support the view that the Childs Fund was parochial: all were Yale men except Peyton Rous, and three of the five, including Rous and Bayne-Jones, were Hopkins-trained. On the NCI, see also Phillips interview, 476–78, and Daniel M. Fox, "The Politics of the NIH Extramural Program, 1937–1950," *Journal of the History of Medicine and Allied Sciences*, XLII (October, 1987), 447–66.

27. Report on Meeting of January 31, 1938, pp. 12–13, in The Jane Coffin Childs Fund for Medical Research: Reports of the Director. In 1939 George M. Smith, an adviser to both the Childs Fund and the Anna Fuller Fund, became a member of the NACC. See *Journal of the National Cancer Institute*, IV (April, 1944), 430.

lected small projects; to provide larger grants to investigators with definite, broad programs already under way; to support a great center of research at Yale; and to coordinate their efforts with outside agencies. This added up to little more than a determination to close no doors. Money spoke louder than words, and the advisers proposed to spend about $222,000 over the next three years, with the lion's share going to Yale. B-J took $10,000 a year for his own laboratory, to get work on viruses started—the most conspicuous gap in the university's cancer program—and lured F. Duran-Reynolds from the Rockefeller Institute to do the research.

In practice the broad principles tended to cancel each other out. Much debate served little purpose but to clear away mental brushwood. The Childs fund would be used primarily (though not uncritically) for Yale, to make the local program as complete as possible. But enough outside grants would be given to satisfy the terms of the donation and to avoid having other foundations pull out of Yale.[28]

As director, B-J became a full-fledged member of the species that has since been designated the Philanthropoid. The American Society for the Control of Cancer elected him a member of the board; the *American Journal of Cancer* appointed him to its editorial board after receiving $5,000 from the Childs fund. He dealt with his opposite numbers at the Rockefeller and Pasteur institutes. He was in on the ground floor of a growth industry. By 1939 he estimated that about $1 million a year was available from all sources for American cancer research. NCI spent about $400,000 a year. Yale alone received between $125,000 and $130,000 from the Childs fund, the Anna Fuller Fund, the International Cancer Research Foundation, the Finney-Howell Research Foundation, the National Research Council, and the Hubbard-McCormick Clinical Cancer Research Fund. A round of meetings and conferences kept B-J on the road several months of every year and taught him most of what was to be known about current trends in research.[29]

Thus in 1939 he conferred with Eugene L. Opie of Cornell Medical College in New York City about his work on leukemia, and with

28. Report on Meeting of January 31, 1938, pp. 19–20, 23–24, 36; Phillips interview, 468. Such research reflected the influence of Rous, who first identified a filterable virus as the cause of an avian cancer.
29. Report of June 1, 1938, p. 35.

Robert Millikan of the California Institute of Technology on the treatment of cancers by X rays. From August through November of 1940 he visited Tulane and Louisiana State University medical schools in New Orleans, noting at Tulane the work of surgeons Alton Ochsner and Michael E. DeBakey in clinical studies of lung cancer. ("Investigators and clinicians in New Orleans are of the definite opinion," B-J reported, "that cancer of the lung is increasing, particularly in males. The cause of this increase is not known.") Back in New Haven he met Joseph Needham, the English embryologist and future historian of civilization and science in China; in Boston he spent some time with Shields Warren, later chief medical officer of the Atomic Energy Commission and a leader in radiation medicine; and in Bethesda, Maryland, he attended a meeting on cancer at the National Institutes of Health.

At Yale he consulted visiting Harold C. Urey, already a Nobel Prize winner, about his work on the use of radioactive isotopes as chemical tracers in the body. In Chicago he saw an experiment that he might have connected with the Ochsner and DeBakey observations, but apparently did not. A doctor "demonstrated rabbits on whose ears he had produced papillomatous growths [*i.e.*, benign tumors] by the application of tobacco tar from pipes."[30]

Yet over the urgent work of many excellent minds a new shadow had begun to fall. Even as American cancer research began its first period of vigorous growth, the war in Europe was overtaking it. And the war would make its own demands on the country's medical researchers. Well aware of what impended, B-J reported in November, 1940, that he expected cancer research to be "disorganized" by military needs. Times of emergency stimulate applied science but seldom basic research. The rule held especially true for cancer. Cancer was not a military disease and could hardly compete with the immediate need for new methods to combat infection and trauma. Doctors would be pulled into the military, research funds diverted, laboratories set to other tasks; in 1940, NCI's research program was curtailed, and by early 1942 its grants had almost ceased.[31]

30. The Jane Coffin Childs Memorial Fund for Medical Research: Reports of Director, 1940–1943, Vol. II, 100–103.

31. Report of November 18, 1940, 113; see also Fox, "NIH Extramural Program," 452. In the postwar period, of course, national funding for research drastically reduced the relative

In 1940 B-J was a former master, a former dean, an important man in a field that wartime needs would soon shoulder aside. To his credit, he showed little concern with personal disappointments. The rush of events did not encourage dwelling on private sorrows.

Instead, his old patriotism and taste for action sharpened as calamity engulfed the world. In his last year as master of Trumbull, the Munich crisis had found him arguing against his students, who were still repeating the slogans of a pacifism that events had overtaken. War in Poland followed in September, 1939, bringing B-J a sense of "great objects moving in the dark." The fall of France, the evacuation of Dunkirk, and the opening rounds of the Battle of Britain soon followed. Deeply moved, B-J listened to Edward R. Murrow's broadcasts from wartime London, which "inspired and kept ablaze" his sense of inherited loyalties to England and France.

Refugee children showed up in the faculty houses. Rearmament began, and in April, 1940, the Yale Corporation gave approval for the affiliation of the School of Medicine with U.S. Army Surgical Hospital No. 39. Under this arrangement, the school supplied doctors and volunteer nurses, while the government provided the hospital's commander—usually a career medical officer well versed in Army ways—plus enlisted component, equipment, and physical plant. But the four-hundred-bed surgical hospital was unduly limited for an institution the size of Yale, and the board of New Haven Hospital soon suggested a one-thousand-bed general hospital unit instead.[32]

B-J had resumed his membership in the Medical Corps reserve during the 1920s, and by 1939 he had attained the rank of lieutenant colonel despite no apparent participation in formal training. The connection made him a natural go-between. In June, 1940, he traveled to Washington to present Yale's request to Maj. Gen. James C. Magee, surgeon general of the army, who invited the university to make a formal proposal. Yale's affiliation with the 19th General Hospital followed

---

significance of private foundations, including the Childs Fund. See Phillips interview, 483. See also Fielding L. Garrison, *An Introduction to the History of Medicine* (Philadelphia, 1929), 790, and Shryock, *American Medical Research*, 275.

32. Phillips interview, 511–12.

on September 26, 1940. Now fifty-one years old, B-J did not join the unit he had helped to form; after a roller-coaster ride of successes and disappointments, his future as the war began seemed nearly as unpredictable as the world's.[33]

33. Bayne-Jones to Seymour, June 14, 1940, Seymour to Magee, June 27, 1940, Magee to Seymour, June 27 and July 9, 1940, Maj. Gen. E. S. Adams, The Adjutant General, to Seymour, September 26, 1940, all in C-39(3), Box 16, SBJC. See also DA Form 66, Record of Service, in Bayne-Jones's Personnel (201) File, Federal Personnel Records Center, St. Louis. The fact that Bayne-Jones not only remained a reserve officer but continued to rise in rank probably reflected his rising status in the medical world; the army medical department wanted to stay in contact with him.

EIGHT

Save and Slay

Toward the end of December, 1940, the army's surgeon general sent the adjutant general a letter that changed B-J's life. A few months earlier, Congress had enacted the nation's first peacetime draft. Few human populations are more susceptible to disease than young soldiers, living among crowds of strangers under the stress of basic training. Noting that camp ailments had already "reached epidemic proportions" and alarmed about the chances for a new influenza epidemic, Maj. Gen. James C. Magee asked permission to appoint a board of civilian experts to keep watch on the spread of disease in the army.[1]

The actual source of the proposal that bore the surgeon general's name was a rising star of the medical department, Lt. Col. James Stevens Simmons. Simmons had come to Washington for a special task. One of the oldest demands laid upon military doctors was that of preventing disease among the troops. Centuries before the germ theory was proven, surgeons of Western armies attempted to enforce a measure of sanitation and cleanliness on the basis of theories that associated disease with offal and waste, through the pollution of the air. The revolution in medicine had brought new insights to the old struggle, and during World War I the sanitation division of the surgeon general's office had acted as a health department for the army.

But the budgets of the interwar years had reduced the size of the army, and the end of the draft had lessened dangers to health caused by the mixing of great masses of men from varied backgrounds. As World War II approached, preventive medicine had no standing as a specialty in the Office of the Surgeon General. Instead, its concerns were "diffused in nameless fashion," said B-J, through the professional services division. Here, jumbled with many others having different concerns, were the officers who received the reports of sanitary inspectors, collected statistics of morbidity and mortality, and sought to control venereal diseases. When the threat of global war pointed up the

---

1. See printed copies in E-15, Box 23, SBJC.

hopeless inadequacy of the situation, Simmons took on the task of organizing preventive medicine.[2]

Simmons was astute, headed for a star in the army and the deanship of Harvard's School of Public Health after he laid the uniform aside. Sometime in the second half of 1940, he and Dean Francis Blake of Yale's School of Medicine drafted a proposal for a board to deal with infectious diseases in the army. They brought influenza into its title as a selling point; the possibility of a new pandemic in the camps was calculated to appall army and national leaders, who remembered the aftermath of World War I. The surgeon general agreed to sign the proposal, the adjutant general endorsed it, and on January 11, 1941, the secretary of war established the Board for the Investigation and Control of Influenza and Other Epidemic Diseases in the Army. Its unwieldy name caused it to be called, at first unofficially and then officially, the Army Epidemiological Board.[3]

By autumn the board had enrolled an impressive list of civilian medical researchers and had organized its work under a number of subordinate commissions. Blake was president, and under him served representatives of the Rockefeller Institute for Medical Research, the International Health Division of the Rockefeller Foundation, and the Johns Hopkins, Yale, Vanderbilt, and University of Pennsylvania medical schools. These institutions paid the salaries of their members and donated laboratory space for research; the army paid only a twenty-dollar daily consultant's fee to each. The aim was to spot, and if possible to anticipate, epidemic outbreaks and provide expert, on-the-spot examination and recommendations—"fire fighting," board members called it.[4]

2. Annual Report, Preventive Medicine Division (1941), 1, in Office of the Surgeon General: World War II Administrative Records, 1940–1949, Entry 46A, Box 15, RG 112. On the earlier history of preventive medicine in the army, see Bayne-Jones, *The Evolution of Preventive Medicine in the United States Army, 1607–1939* (Washington, 1968).

3. This account largely follows the Phillips interview, 537–39. See also The Adjutant General to Commanding Generals of All Armies, Air Force General Headquarters, Departments, and Corps Areas, March 24, 1941, in E-15, Box 23, SBJC. For convenience, the board will hereafter be referred to as the Epidemiological Board.

4. Memorandum, The Surgeon General to Maj. Gen. R. C. Moore, Deputy Chief of Staff, September 2, 1941, in E-16, Box 23, SBJC; Bayne-Jones, "Board for the Investigation and Control of Influenza and Other Epidemic Diseases in the Army," *Army Medical Bulletin*, No. 64 (October, 1942), 1–22.

Among many names on the board's roster that were already well-known appeared several that only became famous at a later time: Albert B. Sabin was a member of the Commission on Neurotropic Virus Diseases, and Jonas Salk later joined the Commission on Influenza. B-J became director of the Commission on Epidemiological Survey established on February 26, 1941. Still a civilian like his colleagues, through Blake's influence he returned to military preventive medicine for the first time since his long-ago service on the Western Front.[5]

B-J's commission, explained Simmons, would "devote its entire time and facilities to studying the distribution and incidence of disease-producing organisms among troops, with the aim of spotting incipient epidemics . . . *before they occur.*" This was an interesting idea that led in practice to much tedious work. Throat swabs from representative samples of troops were supposed to show a normal distribution of the various organisms that inhabit the healthy body; any sudden increase in a particular group of organisms (*e.g.*, meningococci) might signal an epidemic in the making.

B-J set up his teams (he called them listening posts) in the 1st Corps area near Boston, the 4th Corps in Durham, North Carolina, the 9th Corps in San Francisco, and at San Juan, Puerto Rico. Predictably, members soon lost interest in taking endless throat swabs and became involved in the study of local diseases—in Louisiana, atypical pneumonia among the masses of troops gathered for the great prewar maneuvers, and in California, a fungal infection whose spores, blowing about the Army Air Corps' desert training bases on the dry, dusty winds, caused the southern San Joaquin Valley to be closed to ground-forces training. The Commission on Epidemiological Survey worked on many camp diseases but apparently never predicted an epidemic.[6]

Similarly, the practical work of most commissions failed to follow any set pattern; the work of different commissions overlapped, and some individual researchers pursued a variety of interests. Yet the

5. Minutes of the Board for the Investigation and Control of Influenza and Other Epidemic Diseases in the Army, Third Meeting (June 19, 1941), 2–4, 7, in Armed Forces Epidemiological Board Records, 1941–1963, RG 334, NARA. (These minutes will hereinafter be cited AEB, Minutes.)

6. Col. James S. Simmons, MC, to Harvey H. Bundy, Special Assistant to the Secretary of War, September 22, 1941, in E-16, Box 23, SBJC. See also Phillips interview, 545; AEB, Minutes, Second Meeting (February 6, 1941), 5.

board did pioneering research in many fields, made a number of practical contributions to army medicine, and—perhaps most important of all—provided a model for the military's future role as a patron of civilian medical research in both peace and war. Through the board, B-J took part in shaping that role, not only during the war but for decades after it.

His work for the army grew in other ways as well. By the end of 1941 he had been drawn into the most paradoxical concern of military medicine—biological warfare (BW).

The idea of waging war by deliberately spreading disease has long haunted the human mind. Whether medieval anecdotes of plague victims cast into beleaguered cities by catapults contain any truth remains questionable. BW has provoked widespread skepticism among historians, who find hard evidence of it elusive; among scientists, who know how difficult it is to start an epidemic; and among professional soldiers, who fear weapons they cannot control.

Yet in the twentieth century, enthusiasts for BW have also been common, their numbers increasing as scientists became better able to grow microbes in laboratories. The old aim of starting epidemics gave way to that of causing widespread sickness by saturating enemy-held areas with high concentrations of pathogens. In World War II, all the major combatants except Germany would set up large programs of research, and the Japanese would actually use or attempt to use plague against their Chinese foes.[7]

Among the enthusiasts was Simmons. Like others similarly entranced, he speculated during the thirties on the possibilities of enemy attack with biological weapons. Simmons' favorite idea, based on his service in Panama, was that the Japanese might use yellow fever as a means of attacking the Canal Zone. He seized upon a report that a Japanese had attempted to obtain yellow fever virus from the Rockefeller Foundation by bribery and urged the foundation to prepare yellow fever vaccine for the American garrisons in Hawaii and the Philippines.

7. For bibliography on biological warfare, see footnotes to Albert E. Cowdrey, "'Germ Warfare' and Public Health in the Korean War," *Journal of the History of Medicine and Allied Sciences*, XXXIX (April, 1984), 153–72.

In May, 1941, a report fabricated by "an eccentric and unreliable German refugee scientist" living in Switzerland gave him a new argument: that the Germans were also preparing to use biological weapons. (In fact, German efforts to organize a program were only getting under way at the time, and Hitler soon forbade all work on offensive BW weapons.) The surgeon general expressed skepticism but also began to seek expert advice on "all aspects of offensive and defensive methods and tactics."[8]

Meanwhile, Simmons wrote Harvey H. Bundy, special assistant to the secretary of war, telling him of the report and urging that serious consideration be given to developing facilities within the Medical Department for intensive research on the defensive aspects of BW. Others were also dabbling in the field; research began at Edgewood Arsenal, and the Chemical Warfare Service sought and secured permission to begin the study of offensive aspects of the problem.

On October 1, Secretary of War Henry L. Stimson asked the National Academy of Sciences to set up a civilian advisory committee. The result was the WBC Committee, so called in a stab at secrecy. (The letters BW were simply reversed.) B-J—well known for his government work and his background in bacteriology—became a member, as did the chairman of the National Research Council, the president of the academy, and representatives of the Rockefeller International Health Research Institute and the medical faculties of Johns Hopkins, Cornell, and the University of Chicago. Simmons, Capt. Charles Stephenson—a medical officer from the Navy's Bureau of Medicine and Surgery—and Lt. Col. Tom Whayne of the Preventive Medicine Service were named liaison members of the WBC. During its year of existence (October, 1941, through September, 1942), the WBC also made contact with the similar M-1000 committee in Canada and with the British.[9]

After study, the committee reported that biological warfare was entirely feasible. Its recommendation to "study the possibilities of such warfare from every angle . . . and thereby reduce the likelihood of its use" formed the basis of the nation's program of research. In April,

8. [E. S. Robinson ?], History of the Relation of the Surgeon General's Office to Biological Warfare Activities, in File HD: 314.7–2 (Biological Warfare–History), 17, in Entry 31 (ZI), Box 268, RG 112.

9. Rexmond C. Cochrane, History of the Chemical Warfare Service in World War II (1 July 1940–15 August 1945): Biological Warfare Research in the United States, Vol. I, 6, 14–15, and Vol. II, Appendix A. MS history No. 4-7.1BB, in CMH.

1942, Stimson wrote President Roosevelt: "Biological Warfare is, of course, 'dirty business' but in the light of the [WBC] committee's report, I think we must be prepared. And the matter must be handled with great secrecy as well as great vigor." On May 15, 1942, Roosevelt approved the creation of a biological warfare research organization.[10]

The launching of the effort was somewhat marred by the skepticism of the Army General Staff, which urged that the whole matter be turned over to a civilian agency. Paul V. McNutt's Federal Security Agency became its repository for a time, establishing the War Research Service under Merck & Company's George W. Merck, an ardent supporter of the program. Here, too, B-J served as a consultant from August, 1942, to June, 1944. Harvey Bundy of the war department and Vice-Admiral Ross T. McIntire, surgeon general of the navy, provided military liaison. When the civilian organization proved unable to direct a huge research and development program, the Chemical Warfare Service captured the endeavor, centralizing direction under the Special Projects Division in the office of its chief.[11]

During the war years the United States invested some forty million dollars in plant and equipment. Laboratories and test facilities sprang up at Camp Detrick, Maryland, conveniently close to the capital, and in the moonscape scenery of Dugway Proving Ground, Utah, on the dry bed of Lake Bonneville, an ancient sea as big as Rhode Island. Testing stations were set up on Grosse Ile in the Saint Lawrence River, where the Canadians soon began the mass production of anthrax, and on Horn Island, a sandy strip of dunes and marshes off the Mississippi gulf coast, not far from the Denegres' summer refuge, Malua. A production facility was set up at Vigo, near Terre Haute, Indiana. The navy established a center in Berkeley, California, where scientists experimented with plague as a weapon. Like the Canadians, the army was particularly interested in anthrax, a favorite also of the British pro-

10. "Biological Warfare: Report to the Secretary of War By Mr. George W. Merck, Special Consultant for Biological Warfare," in *U.S. Army Activities in the United States Biological Warfare Programs, 1942–1977* (Washington, 1977), Vol. II, p. A-2; Stimson quotation in Robert Harris and Jeremy Paxman, *A Higher Form of Killing: The Secret Story of Chemical and Biological Warfare* (New York, 1982), 95–96. See also Robinson, History, 42.

11. George W. Merck, "Biological Warfare," *Journal of the American Pharmaceutical Association*, VII (July, 1946), 301–10; Cochrane, History of Chemical Warfare Service, Vol. I, 7; Robinson, History, 50.

gram at Porton, England. But the army also carried out studies on a variety of other diseases affecting humans, animals, and crops; and a joint American-Canadian commission studied animal diseases at Harvard and elsewhere.

American volunteers at Dugway were infected experimentally with Q fever, a rickettsial disease whose symptoms mimicked primary atypical pneumonia. Bombs were produced that burst "into little round packages," said B-J, "that flutter away and scatter the stuff, bombs that produce smoke-like emulsions in the air that drift over fields." Studies of aerosols were particularly intense. Army experimenters worked out the exact size of droplets that would penetrate the lungs most deeply, in studies that yielded a wealth of information on the airborne transmission of disease. Meanwhile, the British exploded anthrax bombs near tethered sheep, and the Japanese did the same to human beings—Chinese, Russian, and Korean prisoners—in their experimental facility at Pingfan, near Harbin, Manchuria.[12]

In the growing American endeavor—a smaller, cheaper Manhattan project whose miracle weapons were never put to use—the army medical department functioned mainly as observer, consultant, and specialist in defense against enemy BW attacks. Responsibility went chiefly to the Special Protection Unit in Simmons' Preventive Medicine Service. For a time in 1942, General Marshall became a believer, ordering the army's Hawaiian Department to embark on an elaborate program of defensive measures. Later in the war, a toxoid intended to protect against botulism would be rushed to England, but it would never be used by the Allied troops training to invade Europe. In prisoner-of-war camps, medics drew blood from German soldiers in an effort to discover if the enemy had inoculated his own troops as a prelude to attacking Allied soldiers.

Medical attitudes toward germ warfare combined moral disapprobation, scientific skepticism, and professional interest. B-J embodied the whole range of fascination and doubt. Years afterward, he called the program that he had helped to launch "all very interesting, and as alarming as you want to make it, and as foolish as you want to make it." Noting that "the philosophical and moral problems were very difficult

12. Phillips interview, 520. The Japanese experiments have received widespread attention. See Cowdrey, "'Germ Warfare,'" 155, and sources cited there.

of solution," he endorsed the old-fashioned medical ethics of the wartime surgeon generals: "I'm sure General Magee and Major General Norman T. Kirk, his successor, couldn't bear the thought of the medical department going into biological warfare and killing people in what they thought was a very dirty and sneaky method." Yet in wartime no possible enemy move could be overlooked, and in adopting the defensive side of BW as its own, the medical department, as future events were to show, set its feet upon a slippery slope.[13]

For the American army, fear of BW helped to produce immediate effects that were both unintended and unfortunate. Faced with impending operations in tropical zones and believing in the possibility of Japanese germ attacks, Simmons, according to B-J, "used this [BW] scare to persuade the general staff and others to sanction vaccination of American soldiers against yellow fever." (In fact, the danger of BW seems to have been only one of several considerations in setting the program in motion, and not the most important.) In any case, immunizations began in the late fall of 1941. But the following February an epidemic of what was then called homologous serum jaundice—hepatitis B, to a later generation—broke out among American troops around the world. At a time when American forces faced overwhelming odds in the Pacific, more than 2,400 men were laid low in Australia and another 2,400 in Hawaii; Lt. Gen. Joseph G. Stilwell fell ill in Burma.

In the same month, B-J put on his uniform again, at Simmons' invitation, and came to Washington. Soon he found himself deeply involved in seeking the cause of what had become a major scare to the army staff. Skillful work by the Epidemiological Board and the Public Health Service demonstrated that the geographical distribution of cases coincided with certain lot numbers of yellow fever vaccine prepared by the Rockefeller Foundation. The disease had been caused by contaminated serum. In this roundabout way, the only worldwide epidemic to strike the army during the war—resulting in some 49,000 cases and 84 deaths—could be traced at least in part to American leaders' belief in the possibilities of biological warfare.[14]

13. Phillips interview, 515–27.

14. Phillips interview, 516, 523, 546–47; Bayne-Jones, "The Outbreak of Jaundice in the Army," Circular Letter No. 95, Surgeon General's Office, reprinted in *Journal of the American Medical Association*, CXX (1942), 51–53; John P. Paul and Horace T. Gardner,

B-J's decision to accept Simmons' invitation to join the Preventive Medicine Division had been quick; he had taken only one day to make up his mind. He retained his faculty status at Yale, and continued to work for the Childs fund, editing its journal for a time on the top of a footlocker in a tiny hotel room. An industrious plodder at the medical school was appointed his assistant, and throughout the war years paid monthly visits to the capital, carrying an enormous briefcase full of grant applications for B-J to review. [15]

But this was merely B-J's overtime. His work for the army filled his days and rapidly grew to fascinate him. The mission of Simmons' office lay close to public health and remote from conventional medicine. As in World War I, B-J was obliged to reorient his own thinking to meet the needs of "the public health of the community of the Army." Though B-J claimed a continuing interest in preventive medicine (tying it, as he did with most things, to his family through Gorgas) in most respects he had drifted far away from it as dean at Yale. Despite his bows to the visions of Winternitz, Angell, and Winslow, he had attuned himself to the conventional view that the business of medicine is disease, not health; his one major effort in the preventive field, the Institute of Nutrition, had been frustrated.

But the army did not permit him to follow the conventional line. In the civilian world the practitioner usually was consulted only by the sick and earned his bread entirely by serving them. In the military, the doctor received board, lodging, and a salary for performing various duties, some medical and some soldierly. Perhaps his most important was to keep his men well and ready to fight. As B-J said, "The striking power of an army is dependent upon the number of physically fit troops available for duty," not upon the number being scientifically cared for

"Viral Hepatitis," *Preventive Medicine in World War II: Communicable Diseases Transmitted Through Contact or by Unknown Means* (Washington, 1960), 419–32; Arthur P. Long, "The Army Immunization Program," *Preventive Medicine in World War II: Personal Health Measures and Immunization* (Washington, 1955), 306–309; J. Austin Kerr, "The Clinical Aspects and Diagnosis of Yellow Fever," in *Yellow Fever*, ed. George K. Strode (New York, 1951), 423. The vaccine was administered to troops en masse because no one could tell where a particular man might be sent. Hence the outbreak appeared in all theaters.

15. On Bayne-Jones's transition to Washington, see Phillips interview, 615–16, 811–12.

in hospitals. Indeed, an ideally successful military physician might never see a sick man at all.[16]

Simmons' vision extended far beyond the confines of the surgeon general's domain. A military Winslow or Winternitz, he saw relationships everywhere, emphasized the social and interconnected character of medicine, and built his bureaucratic kingdom upon it. Within the army, preventive medicine required concerted action among medics, line officers, and the quartermaster corps, which provided the army with shoes, clothing, food, equipment, and bathing facilities. But the civilians among whom the soldiers lived and fought must be kept healthy also. Hence preventive medicine contributed in essential ways to the work of civil affairs—the army units that dealt with friendly governments and liberated peoples—and to the work of military government, which ordered the affairs of conquered enemies.

In some ways, the army was the perfect environment for preventive medicine, for military discipline met the problem of enforcing health regulations. Yet preventive medicine was notably unspectacular: if it succeeded, by definition nothing happened. Hence it was easy to denigrate or to ignore. During times of peace its lessons for wartime were quickly forgotten, as the United States for a variety of reasons forgot the impact that malaria could have on military operations, paying a heavy price in young lives on Bataan, Guadalcanal, and New Guinea during the same months when B-J was learning the ropes in Washington.[17]

Hence the importance of a man like Simmons. B-J called him "a preventive medicine evangelist," a man of burning enthusiasms and no less fiery ambitions. By nature kind, "a lovable person," he was also high-strung, well aware of his own brains, and impatient of stupidity—another of those hot natures, like Zinsser's, with whom B-J's cool objectivity and humor worked so well. Luckily for the army, Simmons' skills as an empire builder were formidable, and the organization he put together was lean and practical.

16. Bayne-Jones, Memo on Preventive Medicine for The Surgeon General's Use in Hearings Before the Subcommittee of the Committee on Appropriations, House of Representatives, May 2, 1942, p. 3, in File No. 319.1–2 (Preventive Medicine Division) SGO Calendar Year 1941, RG 112.

17. Bayne-Jones, *Evolution of Preventive Medicine*, 1, 2–3.

Starting in 1940 with only two like-minded officers, he built within the surgeon general's office an organization of large and elastic functions. By 1942 his office had six branches. Epidemiology ran the army's entire immunization program, organized a belated but effective antimalaria program, and worked in tandem with the Epidemiological Board. Occupational Hygiene oversaw the health of 730,000 workers in the more than five hundred arsenals, industrial plants, and ports of embarkation then run by the army. Sanitation, among many other duties, pursued the development of new insecticides and introduced the Halazone water-purification tablet and the freon-powered aerosol "bomb." Sanitary Engineering worked with the Public Health Service to suppress malaria around training camps in the southern United States. Venereal Disease Control led the army's ultimately successful fight against this occupational disease of soldiers. Laboratories Branch exercised "advisory supervision" over medical department laboratories, and established the Armored Force Medical Research Laboratory at Fort Knox to study the medical consequences of tank warfare. In time, Simmons set up his own civil affairs branch, under Col. Thomas B. Turner, a Johns Hopkins doctor who had treated and counseled Nan during her troubles in 1929.[18]

Another man recruited early by Simmons—always "his own best personnel officer"—was his friend and fellow regular army medical officer, Lt. Col. Leon A. Fox. Starchy Col. Tom Whayne judged him "an arrogant, superficial, lively, articulate mountebank," and a "'bright damfool.'" Intelligent, impulsive, and often picturesque in language, Fox was an original nature in a conformist army, for whom the surgeon general had some difficulty in finding suitable assignments. But B-J was to find in him a useful colleague in his own most important wartime endeavor.[19]

18. Preventive Medicine Division, Annual Report, July 1, 1942–June 30, 1943, pp. 3–12, in Box 17, SGO: World War II Administrative Records, RG 112; Whayne, Memo on Subdivision of Medical Intelligence (1941), April 27, 1942, in Box 15, *ibid*. See also Phillips interview, 619–20. Turner, a bacteriologist, took part in the BW organization, served on OSRD's Medical Research Committee, and later became dean of the Johns Hopkins University Medical School.

19. Phillips interview, 621–22. Whayne quotation in his Critique of Manuscript *War and Healing*, January, 1989, p. 3, in the author's collection.

By early 1944, Preventive Medicine had ten subdivisions, more than fifty officers, and a hundred or so clerks. Simmons' hand reached outside the army as well. He used B-J not only as an administrator but for his contacts in government and private medicine—as he used Blake's, and his own. The division's closest contacts were with the committees on medical research maintained by the National Research Council and by Vannevar Bush's Office of Scientific Research and Development; with the navy's Bureau of Medicine and Surgery; with the Public Health Service; with the International Health Service of the Rockefeller Foundation; and with a variety of scientific societies in the fields of biology, medicine, and public health. Anyone in those organizations whom Simmons and Blake did not know, B-J probably did, and he contributed to his office the decades of acquaintanceships he had formed during his work in research, teaching, and receiving and granting foundation funds.[20]

Most of B-J's time, however, went to the work of administration. Simmons was a big-picture man, impatient of detail, and often absent on inspection trips around the world. His genius in selecting subordinates had never showed to better advantage than in his choice of B-J. Simmons' imagination needed curbing, his enthusiasms required cooling. B-J carried into his administrative work the habits of the laboratory, with its unforgiving demand for exactness in all things; among his many official functions was the unofficial but essential one of bringing his chief face to face with the facts. In running the service, B-J was above all things meticulous, and he had the rare ability to master the details of day-to-day operation without preempting his subordinates' duties or losing his grasp of overall policy.[21]

While his responsibilities extended over the whole field of Simmons' operations, there were certain areas in which he took a more personal hand. Blake's Army Epidemiological Board evolved into a sort of brain trust for the Preventive Medicine Service. As a uniformed officer, B-J

20. Phillips interview, 618–19.
21. Interview, Cowdrey with Thomas B. Turner, Johns Hopkins Medical School, May 29, 1987, in author's collection.

no longer headed a commission. Instead he became the board's administrator, the essential personal link between the board and the Preventive Medicine Division, and more generally between the board and the army. He helped to shore up its often perilous finances, persuading hidebound war-department auditors to follow the standards devised by Vannevar Bush's Office of Scientific Research and Development, of which Simmons was a member.

The basic problem was the unpredictability of research and the impossibility of defining its outcome: what, precisely, was the government paying for when it contracted with a university to explore some problem in its laboratories? As B-J acknowledged, "You can't be sure how you're going to come out, and you can't be sure that the problem remains the same while you're working on it." Much slow and patient diplomacy was needed to convince bureaucrats that the government could contract for brains as well as hardware and could legally use the traditionally narrow device of the contract to do the work of a grant, paying for investigations whose ends none could foresee.

Wartime patriotism, however, made many things possible. Universities took on a financial burden by paying salaries and other costs of research. Civilian consultants were dispatched to remote parts of the world, while their pay vouchers traveled almost as far through the tangled jungles of Washington red tape. By future standards the amount expended by the government for advice from the best American medical experts was absurdly small. Between 1941 and 1946 the ten commissions of the Epidemiological Board spent a total of less than $1.5 million.[22]

In dealing with the board and its commissions, B-J functioned in many ways as if he were still a dean. He helped to set the researchers' problems and secured them funding. The results were constructive all around. The army gained access to the laboratories and expertise of academic medical science. The board scientists gained intriguing problems to pursue, funding, and a vast number of experimental subjects. Meanwhile the growing Preventive Medicine Division (or Service, as it

22. Phillips interview, 559; see also Bayne-Jones's remarks in AEB, 10th Meeting, April 26–27, 1945, pp. 2–3, in E-20(1), Box 24, SBJC. On the OSRD, see Irving Stewart, *Organizing Scientific Research for War: The Administrative History of the Office of Scientific Research and Development* (Boston, 1948).

became permanently on January 1, 1944) labored to turn the board's ideas and discoveries into systems and commands.[23]

As he gained experience, B-J throve in the Washington environment. He felt closest to the civilian doctors, of whom he remained one at heart, and was not above feeling scorn for "the standpat Medical Department officers." Yet he respected many of the regulars, too, developing a rapport with Simmons so close that their subordinates automatically assumed that to hear one speak was to know the mind of the other. B-J won the respect of the professional soldiers by his excellent World War I record—displayed in the ribbons he wore on his chest— and grew to like many and admire some of them. He was, in short, back in his natural element, reconciling the Baynes with the Joneses.[24]

Most men would have found these duties enough. But B-J's main contribution to the war effort lay in a different though closely related field: he carried on Zinsser's war against typhus by means Zinsser had never imagined.

In one of his essays, B-J described vividly the course of the disease: The rickettsiae that cause typhus—microbes smaller than bacteria but larger than viruses—invade and destroy the layer of cells that lines the blood vessels, causing many large and small hemorrhages and affecting the action of the heart. The rash that typifies the disease results from vascular lesions in the skin, and the stupor or dementia of victims from similar damage to the brain. Related organisms cause murine typhus, a disease of rodents sometimes spread by fleas to man, the scrub typhus of Asia and some Pacific islands, and American Rocky Mountain spotted fever—among many other ills.

But epidemic louse-borne typhus had by far the deadliest record. During and after World War I, the disease had flared along the whole Eastern front. According to the League of Nations, Serbia (where Zinsser had worked as an agent of the International Red Cross) suffered

23. AEB, Annual Report (1943), 11; Statement by Brigadier General S. Bayne-Jones, USA, Deputy Chief, Preventive Medicine Service, Office of the Surgeon General, U.S. Army, and Director, United States of America Typhus Commission, 7, 9, in E-19(4), Box 23, SBJC.

24. Phillips interview, 556–58.

135,000 deaths in a population of only 2.5 million. Rumania lost several hundred thousand of its 7.5 million inhabitants. Poland was devastated; a quarter of Russia's population may have become ill—some 25 million cases—and 3 million Poles and Russians may have died. Only German success in controlling the disease among its own troops had prevented typhus from spreading to the louse-infested trenches of the Western Front.[25]

World War II seemed likely to bring a reprise. The Germans introduced typhus into their homeland by importing prisoners of war and slave laborers from Eastern Europe. After a decade's absence, the disease reentered Italy, either with Albanian workers or with Italian troops returning from war in the Balkans. In Japan, typhus was endemic among imported Korean miners. During 1942, outbreaks flared throughout North Africa and the Middle East. As Simmons began to examine the problem in the early days of the war, the difficulties the army faced in combating typhus became evident.

In 1942, no known drug killed rickettsiae in the body. Killing lice was possible, of course, but under wartime conditions hard to carry out effectively. People had to strip and bathe while their clothes were steamed. Steam had no residual action; let a soldier return to an infested bunker or a civilian to an infested house, and within twenty-four hours the job had to be done again. Insecticides that killed living lice were either dangerous to humans or failed to destroy the insects' eggs. In talking over typhus with Capt. Charles S. Stephenson of the navy's Bureau of Medicine and Health and Rolla E. Dryer, head of the National Institutes of Health, Simmons reached the conclusion that another commission of experts was needed, representing all three of the uniformed medical services.

He followed precisely the same course he had in creating the Epidemiological Board: He drafted a letter setting out the problem to Chief

25. Zinsser, *Rats, Lice and History*, 229–39; Yves M. Biraud, "The Present Menace of Typhus Fever in Europe and the Means of Combating It," *Bulletin of the Health Organization of the League of Nations*, X (1942–43), 3; Richard P. Strong, George Shattuck, *et al.*, *Typhus Fever with Particular Reference to the Serbian Epidemic* (Cambridge, Mass., 1920); Bayne-Jones, "Typhus Fevers," in *Communicable Diseases*, ed. Ebbe Curtis Hoff, (Washington, 1964), 176–79, Vol. VII of Hoff, ed., *Preventive Medicine in World War II*; Gaines M. Foster, "Typhus Disaster in the Wake of War: The American Polish Relief Expedition, 1919–1920," *Bulletin of the History of Medicine*, LV (1981), 221–32.

of Staff General George C. Marshall and persuaded the surgeon general to sign it. After securing approval, he called a conference of the future players in the typhus game, of whom B-J was one, to plan the course of the United States of America Typhus Commission.

Stephenson, chosen to be its director and elevated to rear admiral rank, soon demonstrated bureaucratic skills that transformed and expanded it. Through Vice-Admiral Ross T. McIntire, the surgeon general of the navy and the official White House physician, he secured an executive order that gave the commission direct access to the highest levels of government, military and civil; made it autonomous within the medical establishments of the army and navy; and allowed it to establish its own channels of communication. The order even provided for a special medal to be issued to those who aided its work, causing a new disease that Fox named "Typhus medalitis"—the urge felt by anyone who killed a louse to acquire the decoration.[26]

The commission emerged from the Oval Office as a bureaucratic *tour de force*. Whether it would perform any useful work remained to be seen. Events soon demonstrated that its best chances of success came from outside, its main threat of failure from within.

It did not lack for weapons. The basic facts of the disease—the rickettsial agent and the louse vector—were known, and the 1930s had brought major advances in the development of an effective vaccine. Zinsser espoused a method of growing rickettsiae using solid agar; other researchers infected mice by blowing rickettsiae into their noses and made a useful vaccine from their lungs, where the parasites grew abundantly. Herald R. Cox of the Public Health Service's Rocky Mountain Laboratories prepared a vaccine using vast numbers of rickettsiae grown in fertilized eggs. In January, 1942, the war department ordered

26. Simmons to Magee, August 5, 1942, and Magee to Chief of Staff, August 5, 1942, cited in Bayne-Jones, "The United States of America Typhus Commission," *Army Medical Bulletin* No. 68 (July, 1943), 8; Bayne-Jones, Memo for File, October 1, 1942, Simmons, Memo for File, October 22, 1942 (signed "J. S. S."), Stimson to Harold D. Smith, December 18, 1942, all in Folder IA, Box 1, Records related to the organization, administration, and policy of the U.S.A. Typhus Commission, RG 112, NARA. See also Fox to Bayne-Jones, March 27, 1945, in Folder March–April, 1945, in United States of America Typhus Commission Papers, NLM.

all troops bound for Asia, Africa, or Europe to be immunized with the Cox-type vaccine. Meanwhile, methods of killing lice improved; a louse powder called MYL was developed, and DDT, its powers discovered by a Swiss firm, began to prove itself in a Department of Agriculture laboratory.[27]

Yet within a short time the success and even the rationale of the commission were in doubt. In November, 1942, American and British troops invaded French Northwest Africa. Here the army discovered typhus beyond Simmons' worst imaginings. Throughout the year, one of the most severe epidemics since the end of World War I had raged in the precise region where the Allies landed—more than 77,000 recorded cases and perhaps 500,000 more that went unreported. And here the first American victory over typhus was won without help from the commission. American troops moved among the local population, fought battles, lived in the field, picked up lice, and as opportunity permitted pursued sex—often with success, to judge by the incidence of venereal disease.

But very few caught typhus and none died. The disease was so rare in the United States that few men could have been naturally immune. At a stroke, the problem of epidemic typhus ceased to be a concern of the field forces and instead became a matter for Civil Affairs and Military Government. Those in danger were not the troops—immunized by the Cox vaccine—but the tens of millions of civilians in the war zone, who could neither be immunized en masse nor subjected to effective health discipline.[28]

With much of its supposed mission lost, the commission quickly developed internal problems that seemed to threaten the rest. A small group of strong personalities—soldiers, sailors, Public Health Service

27. H. R. Cox and J. E. Bell, "Epidemic and Endemic Typhus: Protective Value for Guinea Pigs of Vaccine Prepared from Infected Tissues of the Developing Chick Embryo," *Public Health Reports*, LV (1940), 110. A useful survey of the various techniques and their problems is John P. Fox, "Immunization Against Epidemic Typhus," *American Journal of Tropical Medicine and Hygiene*, V (May, 1956), 464–79.

28. G. Grenoilleau, "L'Epidemie de typhus en Algerie (1941–1942–1943)," *Archives de l'Institut Pasteur d'Algerie*, XXII (December, 1944), 353–79; Bayne-Jones, "Typhus Fever," 195, 199; Col. Perrin C. Long to Chief, Preventive Medicine Service, October 10, 1945, A Historical Survey of the Activities of the Section of Preventive Medicine, Office of the Surgeon, MTOUSA [Mediterranean Theater of Operations, U.S. Army], 3 January 1943 to 15 August 1943, USATC Records, RG 112, NARA.

officers, and civilians—the members sometimes seemed almost as interested in fighting one another as in tackling typhus. Stephenson, though a man of personal charm and well respected in the civilian research community, appeared unable either to lead or drive his team except to the accompaniment of grumbling and bitter complaints.

The commission was divided into two echelons, one in Washington and one in the field. In January, 1943, Stephenson and his crew departed for Cairo, Egypt, to begin its fact-finding mission on typhus. The month was not out before disaster struck. Stephenson suffered a heart attack, and shortly afterward another. Simmons hastily selected his old friend Col. Leon A. Fox to take Stephenson's place, secured him a promotion to brigadier general, and dispatched him to Egypt. But Fox, instead of calming the internal squabbles of the commission, joined in them with gusto. Quarrels multiplied between naval and army officers, and especially between the men in uniform and a civilian, the well-known Rockefeller public-health expert, Fred L. Soper. To Simmons Fox gave his prescription: a purge. "Admiral Stephenson— Out!!! . . . Soper—Out!!!!!!"[29]

B-J made haste to meet Fox's demands, reassigning Soper to typhus control work in Algeria. Stephenson, loudly protesting, was shipped home to be retired on medical grounds. Three new members moved into vacated slots on the commission, B-J among them.[30] But internal disorder had left the commission with little to show for its work. In Egypt, it was remote from the American troops in Algeria, isolated in a British-controlled theater. Meanwhile Soper found himself in the middle of things, with a four-man Rockefeller team under him, and with an ally in General Eisenhower's chief of preventive medicine. Soper's mission was to find a way to protect civilians against typhus. Pondering the problem, he turned to an idea first tried in Egypt by a

29. Simmons, Memo for Typhus Commission Files, February 1, 1943; Simmons to Lutes, February 2, 1943; Fox to Simmons, May 26, 1943, in Folder November, 1942–May, 1943, USATC Papers, NLM. See also Fox to Simmons, May 11 and 14, 1943, in Folder IB, Box 1; Fox to Simmons, April 1, 11, 14, 1943, all in Folder USATC General, Box 2, USATC Records, RG 112, NARA.

30. Bayne-Jones to Acting Chief of Staff for Operations, Army Service Forces (Attention, Col. W. L. Wilson), May 15 and 24, 1942, in Folder November, 1942–May, 1943, USATC Papers, NLM. Secret Radio CM-IN-12399 (April 21, 1943), ibid.; Lt. Gen. Brehon Somervell, Commanding General, Army Service Forces, to Chief of Staff of the Army, May 25, 1943, ibid.

colleague: use of a mechanical dustgun to spread insecticidal powder. But Soper made a critical improvement. Knowing the difficulty of persuading Moslem women to remove their clothing, he used the gun experimentally to blow powder under the clothes of prisoners at a local jail, without having them strip. And the powder he used was DDT.

The results were striking. Clothing, instead of protecting the lice, held the insecticide close to the body, where its residual killing power continued to work as new generations of lice hatched out. The method was amazingly quick and easy. Mass demonstrations of the dust gun, including the disinfestation of thousands of louse-ridden Axis prisoners, proved the value of one of the most surprising and by far the most constructive weapon of the war. The method, painless and intriguing to the popular mind, gained in popularity as the Algerians realized that after a treatment they could sleep undisturbed by the lice that had been consuming them. DDT began to appear on the North African black market—a good sign, noted Soper.

A few workers with dust guns could now disinfest multitudes. The elaborate machinery of bathing and steaming had been made obsolete. In conjunction with Cox's vaccine, Soper's dust gun using DDT made possible the defeat of typhus in wartime.[31]

Deeply troubled by the commission's failure, Fox worked in his own way to improve things and found an extraordinary solution: he voluntarily gave up the directorship. "In this scheme," he wrote Simmons, "I have deliberately lowered my own importance. I do not care for personal glory if we can just make a success of the Commission." Simmons immediately decided that B-J must be its new head and must run it from Washington. In the course of one eventful day—August 11, 1943—the commission's center of gravity was reversed and B-J charged with forging a workable organization from the shambles.[32]

31. Soper to Fox, September 2, 1943, in Folder June, 1943–November, 1943, USATC Papers, NLM; Office of the Surgeon, Headquarters, NATOUSA, Circular Letter No. 43, November 11, 1943, subject: Typhus Fever Control, *ibid.* Soper's own account is given retrospectively in F. L. Soper, *et al.*, "Louse Powder Studies in North Africa (1943)," *Archives de l'Institut Pasteur d'Algerie*, XXIII (September, 1945), 183–223.

32. Fox to Simmons, July 27, 1943, Bayne-Jones, Memorandum for Record of U.S.A. Typhus Commission, August 10, 1943, subject: Reorganization, Bayne-Jones, same title, Au-

By army standards the new command arrangement was absurd. B-J, still a colonel, gave orders to Fox, a general. Even after B-J received his own star in February, 1944, Fox was senior to him by date of rank. No member of the Regular Army was likely to forget that fact, and B-J sensed the irony that laced Fox's attitude of formal deference. Yet mutual respect soon developed between men of complementary skills, and B-J's extraordinary tact made a success of the system that Fox's impulsive generosity had introduced.

Fox would direct the commission's field operations in Africa and Europe. B-J would try to fit the commission into the military bureaucracy, preserve its independence, and provide it overall guidance and logistical support. His would be the final decisions and the power to command what remained, despite many oddities, a military organization. But among his scientists he would more often function as a diplomat and persuader than as a general. He could not end the commission's self-destructive inner squabbles nor make it fit for the importance of its mission merely by issuing orders.

Rebuilding the commission and securing its position were the first tasks. B-J obtained new men that Fox wanted. He found the organization itself a secure home within the bureaucracy as a miscellaneous activity of the war department, with direct access to the secretary of war. To ensure its members permanent positions, he persuaded G-1, the army staff personnel division, to increase the surgeon general's officer allotment by a number equal to the commission's list and then to assign its members permanently to the surgeon general's office.[33]

With a skilled administrator in Washington and an energetic enthusiast in the field, the commission came to life. In Naples, Fox worked side by side with Soper to halt an outbreak of typhus under conditions—of winter, war, a hungry and crowded population—that would probably have ensured a major epidemic at any previous time in history. Working through Admiral McIntire, he persuaded President Roosevelt to make vaccine freely available to friendly nations in the

gust 11, 1943, all in Folder II, Box 1, USATC Records, RG 112, NARA. The adjutant general issued the reorganization order on August 21.

33. Bayne-Jones, Memorandum for Record of U.S.A. Typhus Commission, October 30, 1943, *ibid.*

Middle East. At his urging the commission gradually took on a coordinating rather than a merely advisory role. During 1944 its activities
spread around the world: into Asia, where it took on scrub typhus, an
often lethal disease spread by mites; into the Balkans with Tito's parti-
sans; into Greece; into liberated France and the first few miles of conquered German territory. Commission workers became familiar figures, and the dust gun and the clouds of DDT part of the wartime scene
wherever the growing throngs of refugees, prisoners, and former inmates of concentration camps faced the threat of typhus.[34]

In the process the commission changed subtly. A collection of
people became a team. B-J's role in the transformation was substantial.
He served as a damper for Fox's rages and an efficient logistician who
kept supplies moving for the worldwide typhus battle. More than an
administrator or a commander, from the center at Washington he became message center, adviser and father figure to the younger men. He
used his position without hesitation to provide small personal advantages for his people—to get information about an ailing spouse, to obtain promotions, and to cut the endless red tape. Realizing the importance of publications to their future careers, he stretched wartime
secrecy regulations about as far as they would go. His letters to his
subordinates were must unusual for official correspondence: peremp-
tory demands for information mingled with newsy, chatty accounts of
Washington doings, technical advances in their special fields, gossip
about other commission members, congratulations on awards, and
praise for work well done.[35]

As usual with preventive medicine, the commission's victory was
marked by the things that did not happen. One was the great European
typhus epidemic of 1945. Conditions seemed ripe, and sixteen thousand cases were recorded in conquered Germany, most among displaced persons and inmates of concentration camps, before medics of
the field forces and the military government detachments, backed by
commission know-how and supplies, put an end to the outbreak. A
similar danger appeared in conquered Japan, where some thirty thou-

34. Bayne-Jones to Dr. Thomas Parran, December 5, 1943, in folder June, 1943–
November, 1943, U.S. Typhus Commission Papers, NLM.
35. See, *e.g.*, Bayne-Jones to Mrs. John C. Snyder, July 19, 1943, and to Cornelius B.
Philip, June 29, 1944, USATC Papers, NLM.

sand cases were recorded before the incipient epidemic was stamped out by Japanese health workers, directed by the Occupation government, and advised and supplied by the commission.

If the evidence of success was negative, so too were the rewards. When the war was over, commission members could reflect upon the throng of onetime enemies who did not get sick or die; the children who were not left orphans; the human possibilities that were not foreclosed. By comparison with the epic destruction of the time, the work of the commission was little noticed and soon forgotten. But it was this work primarily that caused a wartime insider to say, many years later, that B-J had "probably saved more lives than any doctor I ever knew or heard about."[36]

36. Washington *Post*, March 15, 1970.

NINE

Medical Center

Peace returned, bringing celebrations, awards, and ennui. For his achievements in preventive medicine, B-J received the Typhus Commission medal, adorned with the profiles of Zinsser and Charles Nicolle; the Most Excellent Order of the British Empire, degree of Honorary Commander; and the Distinguished Service Medal. Added to his battlefield decorations from World War I, this was an impressive panoply for a citizen soldier.

In turn, he had the satisfaction of passing out lesser awards to his wartime associates at a love feast held in the National Academy of Sciences building on Washington's Mall. To Blake he gave the Medal of Merit; to Sabin and others, the Legion of Merit; and to almost all who had taken a hand in the wartime effort, an array of Medals of Freedom, army commendation ribbons, and certificates of appreciation. Simmons, now dean of the Harvard University School of Public Health, joined Blake in recommending B-J as second director of the board, an appointment he duly received and held for two years.[1]

Less sweet were his prospects outside the government. His position at Yale now held little interest for him. He had tasted a headier drink, and the university life now struck him as "semi-interment." Nevertheless, he resumed his academic job in 1946, and he and Nan moved some of their belongings to New Haven. He felt anew the peculiar listlessness of the soldier suddenly returned to the tasks of peace. "There is a momentum of Army ways and associations!" he wrote a friend in Washington. "I feel as if I had been away a long time—and miss all of you very much." From time to time he staged reunions for the typhus commission staff, a man dissatisfied with the

---

1. 14th Meeting of the Board, April 15–16, 1946, pp. 2, 8, in E-20(1), Box 24, SBJC. On the OBE award, see materials in I-45, Box 48, *ibid.*, and on the DSM, materials in E-24(T–Z), Box 24, *ibid.* Bayne-Jones's separation from the army is formally given in Maj. Gen. Edward F. Witsell, The Adjutant General, to B-J, May 13, 1946, in E-24(T–Z), Box 24, *ibid.* Bayne-Jones's peacetime work for the Epidemiological Board is treated in Chapter 10.

present, clinging to odds and ends of the past, and uncertain what the future might bring.[2]

In this doleful period sickness struck. The first (and worst) news came from Chicago, where his old friend and sometime roommate Pat O'Brien was diagnosed with cancer. B-J flew to Chicago; Pat's wife and daughter met him at the airport, and he spent that evening and part of the next morning at the sick man's bedside. Yet aside from sympathy, B-J had nothing to offer but expert opinions that confirmed the verdict of Pat's own doctors. Treatments were painful and hopeless. "Science is wonderful," Pat wrote, "but I sometimes envy my ancestors who died too early to know how painfully life can be prolonged."

Restless, the Bayne-Joneses moved to New York, subletting Ruth Zinsser's apartment on 52nd Street. Then Nan fell ill. Bouts of severe pain led in March to gall-bladder surgery that kept B-J at her side whenever he was not drawn away by work to New Haven or Washington. By summer she had recovered; by autumn Pat was dead.[3]

Meanwhile a new and unexpected opportunity had opened for B-J by courtesy of the Cushing family. At Yale the Bayne-Joneses had come to know the great neurosurgeon and his three remarkable daughters. One had married John Hay "Jock" Whitney, an exceedingly rich man. When Whitney needed a seasoned medical administrator and educator for one of his charitable interests she mentioned B-J's name. Shortly thereafter Whitney invited him to lunch at the Knickerbocker Club, to discuss the problems of the New York Hospital–Cornell Medical College Association.

One of the city's great private institutions of healing, the hospital had survived many troubles since King George III had granted its charter. Early in the twentieth century it formed a tentative association with

2. Phillips interview, 829; Bayne-Jones to Captain Waring, June 9, 1946, in Folder May–July, 1946, USATC Papers, NLM.

3. Frederick Christopher to Bayne-Jones, November 12, 1946, Evanston Hospital Association: Report of Pathological Specimen, Bayne-Jones to Christopher, November 16, 1936, all in A-32, Box 7, SBJC. Quotation in *Time* (October 13, 1947), 83–84. O'Brien had become a well-known columnist on a Chicago newspaper, and his frank writing about his illness drew national attention.

Cornell Medical College, and in 1927 both institutions relocated to the bank of the East River, where they occupied an incongruous cluster of shining towers, laboratories, classrooms, brick power stations, and wooden barracks. In the 1930s, Memorial Hospital, where Zinsser had died, affiliated with the medical college and moved across the street. In 1945, Alfred P. Sloan, Jr., General Motors' chairman, and Charles F. Kettering, vice-president and manager of the auto giant's research laboratory, provided four million dollars to create, intimately associated with Memorial, the Sloan-Kettering Institute for cancer research.

The parts of this extraordinary complex (made still more extraordinary by the presence next door of the Rockefeller Institute) were linked by legal bonds whose intricacy and indefiniteness recalled the Holy Roman Empire. Each part remained highly individual, with its own dominant personalities and institutional needs. The financial power of the Whitneys, Hapsburg-like, pervaded the Association and made its concerns a family tradition, if not quite an heirloom. In the 1940s, the problems that Jock Whitney faced were rising costs, a persistent and increasing deficit in the hospital, and an uneasy relationship between the hospital and the college.[4]

On all these matters, B-J—remembering the frictions between the Yale School of Medicine and the New Haven Hospital—had much to offer. As meeting followed meeting, he learned the basic facts of governance at New York Hospital–Cornell. Over the Association reigned (but seldom ruled) a joint administrative board of seven members drawn from the hospital and the medical college. For years the board had been without a chief administrative officer; this, in agreement with Cornell University, Whitney now proposed to supply.

The wooing proceeded in the rosy tradition of such courtships, when promises rise to the lips like smiles. Assurances of freedom, support, and no interference came from Whitney partner William Harding Jackson, who headed the hospital's board of governors, and from President Edmund Ezra Day of Cornell—the successor of Andrew Dickson White at four removes. Perhaps unaware as yet that his last predecessor

---

4. On the background of the institutions, see L. G. Payson to John Hay Whitney, October 27, 1949, in Folder 6, Box 13, Secretary Treasurer, Society of The New York Hospital, Papers (BTFs), 1911–1960, in MANY. See also Morris Bishop, *A History of Cornell* (Ithaca, 1962), 317–21.

had left the organization a bitter man, defeated by its internal quarrels, B-J was ready by the end of February to confess himself "definitely interested."[5]

By the end of April, university and hospital had reached agreement with B-J, and on May 20 they formally announced his appointment as president of the board. He took his new job seriously; well aware that it would demand his full time, he resigned from Yale and from the Childs fund, gave up the editorship of *Cancer Research,* and told the Appleton-Century Company to find a new author for the next edition of the *Textbook of Bacteriology.* He stayed on the Army Epidemiological Board, but ceased to be its director. The resignations were easier because the medical center promised to be all his jobs—in medical administration, treatment, research, and education—rolled into one.

During the years in Washington he had helped to direct preventive health care for tens of millions of people scattered over the world. Now he would help to organize health care for all races, kinds, and conditions of people on the world's island, Manhattan.[6]

All began well. On the day the *Times* announced his appointment, he ceased to be merely a respectable member of New York's crowds and became a citizen of some distinction, greeted as a peer by eminent scientists and directors of foundations. His elevation was cheered by past subordinates like Sabin and by past benefactors like Alice Coffin.

Yet the cheers died quickly. B-J's first year turned into an extended hazing. In plain fact, neither of the institutions he was supposed to lead wanted to surrender its own prerogatives and ways of doing things, and both saw him as a threat. The men who had courted him grew chilly. Jackson growled, "My god B-J—when are you going to quit 'learning'

5. Bayne-Jones to Jackson, February 8, 1947, in E-33(1), Box 25, SBJC; see also Jackson to Bayne-Jones, February 20, 1947, *ibid.*; G. Canby Robinson, An Account of My Experiences as Director of the New York Hospital–Cornell Medical College Association, July 16, 1934, 7, in Folder 5, Box 9, Secretary-Treasurer Papers, 1911–1960, MANY, and Eric Larrabee, *The Benevolent and Necessary Institution: The New York Hospital, 1771–1971* (New York, 1971), 321.

6. New York *Times,* May 20, 1947; see also the hospital newsletter, *The Pulse,* IX (August, 1947), 1, 10, in E-33(1), Box 25, SBJC, and Bayne-Jones to Blake, May 22, 1947, in E-33(2), Box 25, SBJC.

and do something important[?]" and Joseph C. Hinsey, the dean of the college, excluded him from a faculty meeting and told Day that he was "defending the University on this front!"[7]

Yet some of the center's leaders were working to make their new president a success. The hospital's able secretary-treasurer, Laurence G. Payson, had already taken the lead in drawing up amendments to the affiliation agreements that defined B-J's new job. The Society of The New York Hospital accepted the changes in January, 1948. At Cornell the process took longer and involved new humiliations. B-J found the internal temperature at the campus where President White had once entertained him little warmer than the wintry exterior. Nevertheless, the university trustees accepted the agreement—they had little choice, except to return the association's problems to square one—and in February Jackson and Day signed for their two organizations.[8]

The amendments formally adopted the title "The New York Hospital–Cornell Medical Center" and made the president the chief executive officer of the Joint Administrative Board, responsible for the overall direction of the center and for recommending policies and programs. He was made a member ex officio of the hospital's Medical Board, of the executive faculty of Cornell's medical college and school of nursing. A catchall item assured him membership as well in any other boards, committees, or faculties that the Joint Administrative Board might afterward create. He was to prepare the annual joint budget and to be responsible for its administration, and the director of the hospital and the deans of the college and the school of nursing were enjoined to consult him on the preparation of their annual budgets as well. He was to represent educational and research interests within the hospital, and to coordinate the work of the college and the school with the operations of the hospital. His salary and expenses were to be borne equally by the hospital and the university.

This was B-J's charter. It wrote him into everything he wanted to be a part of, and prevented anyone from excluding him from anyplace

7. Bayne-Jones, Memorandum for Record, July 8, 1948, pp. 1, 5–6, in E-35(1), Box 25, SBJC.

8. *Ibid.*, 2–3. On Payson's work, see the penciled foolscap sheets signed L. G. P. in Folder 4, Box 18, Secretary Treasurer Papers, 1911–1960, MANY.

he wished to go. The hazing was over, and he must now make good use of the powers he had been granted.[9]

As in the past, his charm did not fail him. Finding him agreeable, reliable, and able, Day and Jackson, the two chief feudatories of B-J's strange kingdom, signaled that they were willing for him to bear some of their burdens. Feeling that he had "gotten past the personal part," he began to grapple with the medical center's problems, both transient and enduring.[10]

The most intractable was the elementary fact that college and hospital were different worlds. Nowhere did the differences show more clearly than in finance. Cornell University demanded that its medical college present a balanced budget, sacrificing staff and equipment if need be. The college attained balance (precariously) through the substantial grants it received for conducting medical research. The "deficits" of the college—in understaffed, inadequately funded departments, and in underpaid, overworked, and pensionless staff—existed in reality but did not show on the balance sheet.

By contrast, the hospital, with its long tradition of charity care, habitually ran large deficits in dollars and cents. Its income came from fees and voluntary contributions, large and small, and it depended on the 475 members of the Society of The New York Hospital, as well as the United Hospital Fund and the Greater New York Fund, charities that resembled the Community Chest. Poor patients in the teaching wards paid at best a small part of the $14.00 a day they cost the hospital. Paying patients in semiprivate rooms paid $14.00, but because of the greater personal care they received they cost the hospital $16.00. Emergency indigent cases cost as much as ward patients, but the city paid the hospital only $4.50 a day to treat them. Overall, 88 percent of the patients did not pay the full cost of their care. In 1947, when B-J

9. Minutes of the Meeting of the Joint Administrative Board of the New York Hospital–Cornell Medical College Association, December 19, 1947, pp. 506–15, in E-36(1), Box 25, SBJC (hereinafter cited as JAB Minutes).

10. Day to Bayne-Jones, August 14, 1948, and Bayne-Jones to Jackson, December 10, 1950, in E-35-(1), Jackson to Bayne-Jones, November 24, 1948, in E-35(2), all in Box 25, SBJC. Jackson resigned from the Joint Administrative Board during November to become deputy director of the newly formed Central Intelligence Agency. See Jackson to Bayne-Jones, November 29, 1950, in E-35(2), Box 25, SBJC.

came aboard, the hospital had a net annual deficit of $175,000, if depre-
ciation was ignored, and about $1 million if it was not.[11]

Low rates and indigent care were not the whole cause of the
problem. The hospital was huge and formidably bureaucratic. A self-
contained town within the metropolis, it treated some 76,000 patients
during 1947. Its organization was riddled with bastions of private privilege, some of which the new president threatened by his mere existence. Arrangements for paying clinical staff members were feudal in
complexity: some might practice in the hospital and draw an unlimited
income from private patients; others were limited in the outside income
they might earn, or were salaried full-timers. Each individual was inclined to defend his own privileges and to envy his neighbors'.[12]

As a result, B-J often looked—probably often felt—like a designated victim pursued by two mobs, his job a matter of staying one jump
ahead of the tar and feathers. (One consequence was a duodenal ulcer,
the only one he ever developed during a lifetime rich in stress.) As
usual, he had no special agenda. He taught himself and gained the confidence of others by taking up the basics first. His early reports to the
executive committee of the hospital's board of governors typically concerned elevators and the heating plant. Then he progressed to doing
liaison work, keeping the different parts of the center aware of one another's viewpoints and needs. He attended every meeting he could, and
like a wise staffer made sure that he always had something of substance
to contribute, however small.

Gradually he developed a method of coordinating center policy
through a shifting network of ad hoc committees on pressing issues.
Usually he sat in as a member ex officio, while the other members,
representing the interested parts of the center, provided the expertise
on particular issues. The system he created demanded endless patience
and time but rewarded him with unrivaled knowledge, and hence influence, over issues that involved the whole center.

In the process his own philosophy emerged. Fundamentally, he

11. See Jackson's report, "The New York Hospital Today: Our Thoughts and Plans for
Its Future," in The Society of The New York Hospital Record (July, 1947), 2–3, in E-35(4),
Box 25, SBJC; and Hinsey to Bayne-Jones, December 7, 1951, in Folder 6, Box 13, Secretary
Treasurer Papers, 1911–1960, MANY.
12. The Society of the New York Hospital Record (June, 1948), 14–15; JAB Minutes,
November 21, 1947, pp. 502–503, 506, in E-36(1), Box 25, SBJC.

thought that the center's bottom line had nothing, or very little, to do with money. What counted was service rendered, patients treated, research ably carried out, and students competently taught. Hence he was at heart uninterested in balancing the budget. When the nurses demanded a forty-hour week, he gave them what they wanted; when the hospital's director suggested reducing the house staff of almost four hundred interns, residents, and assistant residents, B-J evaded the issue and kept the young people at work. "If we cut services we shall lose opportunities, staff, students and influence," he argued. Better to seek to make up the shortfalls with gifts, and with payments from government and health insurers for services rendered.[13]

Programs of expansion were more to his taste. He hoped to affiliate with other hospitals and clinics in the city, a maneuver that promised benefits to all parties through expanded services, merged facilities, and reduced costs. But each merger required a thousand questions of law, financing, and control to be decided; each involved endless negotiations and a myriad of practical difficulties.[14]

Thus the problem of affiliation with the Hospital for Special Surgery dragged on for years, timed to a slow and stately waltz between the Joint Administrative Board and the curiously named New York Society for the Relief of the Ruptured and Crippled, which governed the smaller hospital. By mid-1948 the entire center had become involved. B-J, after viewing with disgust the quarters allotted male students in barracks on the East River, proposed that the New York Hospital receive from Cornell the land where the barracks stood, giving in exchange a site it owned on York Avenue for a new building to house the students. In turn, the hospital turned over the land to the Hospital for Special Surgery, which agreed to build facilities and move there. The gain for the New York Hospital was a functioning orthopedic service.

Left in the cold were the students, for the $2.5 million needed to build them a new residence hall was, as yet, nowhere to be found. But as the date approached for the barracks to be demolished, Dean Hinsey found the solution. A foundation set up by a Cornell graduate of years

13. *The Society of The New York Hospital Record* (June, 1948), 2–5, in E-35(5), Box 25, SBJC; JAB Minutes, September 19, 1947, p. 495, in Box 25, SBJC.

14. JAB Minutes, September 19, 1947, p. 489, and February 20, 1948, p. 526, in E-36(1) and E-36(2), respectively, Box 25, SBJC.

past supplied the money and, pending construction, the hospital loaned Cornell a building it owned as temporary student quarters. "Now the Hospital has a fine tenant," said a member of the Joint Administrative Board, "and the Medical College has room for its students." He might have added: and the whole Center has given a splendid example of cooperative effort.[15]

The old and loose affiliation with Memorial likewise grew during B-J's tenure. But Sloan-Kettering, under its dynamic director, Cornelius P. Rhoads, was transforming the nature of Memorial Hospital. In 1945 Memorial had transferred its research facilities to the institute; in the years that followed, the hospital became what Hinsey called "a facility, a laboratory, for the use of the Sloan-Kettering Institute, with less clinical research and less care of patients not related to the . . . Institute." Wishing to grant degrees as well, Sloan-Kettering in 1949 turned to Cornell University. President Day agreed to an arrangement by which the Institute would become a graduate school or graduate department of Cornell, with the institute's staff as faculty—in effect, a second, if highly specialized, medical school, standing half a block from the first.[16]

To B-J's anger, Hinsey and the College appeared complaisant. ("In my opinion," he said later, "the medical school had to be defended against its own officers.") Fundamentally, he believed that the needs of medical education could be decided neither by a nonmedical institution (Cornell University) nor by a noneducational one (Sloan-Kettering). Yet he wanted a connection with the research powerhouse down the street. At the end of 1949, Whitney suggested that B-J and Hinsey be appointed as negotiators to bring Sloan-Kettering into the Medical Center, but to do so on B-J's terms.[17]

The critical decisions came in a meeting at the Links Club on December 28. B-J, Whitney, Laurance Rockefeller (representing Memorial and Sloan-Kettering), and a gaggle of lawyers reviewed past propos-

15. JAB Minutes, January 18, 1952, pp. 819–20, in E-38(1), January 30, 1953, in E-38(3), April 23, 1948, pp. 548–49, in E-36(2), May 21, 1948, p. 558, in E-36(3), February 20, 1953, p. 901. The 1948 materials are in Box 25 and the later materials in Box 26, SBJC.

16. Hinsey, Report on Memorial–SKI (1959), 2, and Bayne-Jones, Memorandum for Record, November 30, 1949, in Box 10, Presidents, NYH–CMC, Papers 1945–1975.

17. Bayne-Jones to Hinsey, October 13, 1949, in Folder 4, Box 1, Secretary Treasurer Papers, 1911–1960, MANY. See also JAB Minutes, April 23, 1948, p. 547, in E-36(2), June 18, 1948, in E-36(3), both in Box 25, SBJC. See also Phillips interview, 872, 874.

als. Then B-J put forward his own general formula for agreement. Cornell should not establish a second medical school, nor should the Cornell Medical College faculty control appointments at Memorial and Sloan-Kettering. But provision should be made for the closest possible relationship between the two adjoining centers. A draft agreement was drawn up, providing that Sloan-Kettering Institute's teaching function "will be set up as a Division of the Cornell University Medical College"—the first paragraph of a complex treaty designed to maintain the corporate identity of all parties and to permit close cooperation in teaching.[18]

Though he was quick to point out that much work still remained to be done, B-J finished the meeting with his own point of view established. The rest was cleanup work. The joint agreement had to be modified to permit Cornell to enter into the new arrangement, and many verbal changes had to be made by the lawyers. At the end of the process, however, the basics remained intact: the Sloan-Kettering Division of Cornell University Medical College offered graduate training in cancer and its allied diseases, primarily through participation in research. It taught none of the clinical fields, such as surgery or medicine. To those who completed its courses, the university awarded advanced degrees in the basic (preclinical) sciences. The medical college emerged intact and, indeed, strengthened by the brains, resources and prestige of the Institute.[19]

Defending education, promoting unity, and evading the budget crunch as well as he could, B-J labored to impose his own priorities. Preventive medicine was an area that he found especially congenial: after all, it had become his specialty, insofar as he had one. The evolving role of the twentieth-century hospital as a community health center gave him a welcome opportunity both to press the worthwhile ideas of others and to advance his own.

18. JAB Minutes, April 22, 1949, p. 626, in E-36(3), September 23, 1949, in E-37(2), October 31, 1949, in E-37(3), December 16, 1949, pp. 669–670, all in Box 25, SBJC.

19. JAB Minutes, January 20, 1950, 677–79, April 19, 1950, 701–703, both in E-37(3), Box 25, SBJC. See also Bayne-Jones to Cornelis W. deKiewiet, acting President of Cornell University, May 26, 1950, in Folder 12, Box 1, President's papers, 1939–1962, MANY.

The center's primary field of work in preventive medicine was its own neighborhood—the district of midtown Manhattan called York-ville, whose half-million people lived between Central Park and the East River, from 59th to 96th streets. Outreach programs had already begun, in the outpatient department, in a cancer-detection program, and in a program of preventive psychiatry launched in 1950 by the Payne Whitney Clinic. The last sounded like a Winternitz scheme made real, with cooperative work by anthropologists, social workers, public health officers, doctors, and nurses to identify and treat the disturbed. B-J blessed these efforts but directed his own toward two initiatives that were more conventional but equally wide-ranging: comprehensive care and the Vincent Astor Diagnostic Clinic.[20]

Comprehensive care was the brainchild of the hospital's medical board. With B-J's enthusiastic support, fourth-year students were assigned to serve as "family physicians" to the poor, seeing their patients in the hospital's general medical or pediatric clinics, and guiding the rehabilitation of the handicapped. The work did not involve the students directly in solving social problems, but in order to understand, diagnose, and treat the patients, the students had to become intimately aware of how they lived. The result was a kind of tamed social medicine, free of the illusion that poverty and crime could be cured like infections, but free also of the laboratory bias that saw nothing in the patient but the disease. B-J sat on the plan's advisory committee, urged that social scientists be brought in to help teach medical students, and tried to clear away legal and administrative obstacles to success.[21]

The diagnostic clinic, a proposed benefaction by Astor that combined group practice with prevention, caused a donnybrook with organized medicine. The intent was to provide patients with limited funds a complete diagnostic workup for a moderate fixed fee. B-J inherited the issue but gladly took it up as his own. As a conservative innovator, he liked the prospect that patients would pay a fee well within the range

20. Bishop, *History of Cornell*, 578; Marvin K. Opler, "Epidemiological Studies of Mental Illness: Methods and Scope of the Midtown Study in New York," in *Symposium on Preventive and Social Psychiatry* (Washington, n.d.), especially 125; press release on preventive psychiatry, May 6, 1950, in Folder 2, Box 8, Secretary Treasurer Papers, 1911–1960, MANY.

21. Bayne-Jones to Malcolm P. Aldrich, Administrator of the Commonwealth Fund, June 26, 1951, in Folder 9, Box 1, President's Papers, 1945–1975, MANY.

of middle-class pocketbooks; as a practical man, he hoped to cut into the money paid by New Yorkers for the diagnostic services of distant clinics like the Mayo. The medical societies of the five New York boroughs, however, warned that the clinic would "constitute unfair competition with private practitioners" and that fee-setting by the Hospital would be "corporate practice of medicine." During his career, B-J had encountered town-grown rivalries in many forms, but never had he met more unyielding opposition clothed in the customary fig leaf of professional ethics.[22]

B-J began, as usual, by joining the opposition. This was common sense and, in his position, an inevitability as well. As an active member of the Medical Society for the County of New York, he did much work for the society, got to know its members, chaired its committee on public health, and—in the words of its executive secretary—became acquainted with its "inner workings." Yet the society continued to take stands against group practice and against the center for retaining fees earned by full-timers. On the clinic it was intractable. Hence B-J resorted to a legal fiction and a *fait accompli*. Since the term *clinic* implied free service, he adopted the name Vincent Astor Diagnostic Service (VADS) instead. Since AMA guidelines forbade the corporate practice of medicine, B-J assembled a group of doctors within the hospital to run the service, led by Connie Guion, a North Carolina–born woman physician and a leading spirit of the institution to which she had given her life. B-J then ordered the architects to draw plans. Sure of his legal grounds, he ignored further complaints and pushed the project to completion. The VADS opened in temporary quarters on June 3, 1950; today, forty years later, it continues work in the hospital.[23]

In the course of his many projects B-J arrived at a thoroughgoing conception of the center as a focus of community health. When the

22. JAB Minutes, December 19, 1947, p. 506, in E-36(1), February 20, 1948, p. 527, in E-36(2), both in Box 25, SBJC.

23. JAB Minutes, November 19, 1948, p. 593, in E-36(3), Box 25, SBJC; Bayne-Jones to Arthur M. Master, President, Medical Society of the County of New York, June 9, 1951, in E-64, Box 27, *ibid.*; JAB Minutes, November 24, 1950, in E-37(5), Box 25, December 16, 1949, p. 672, in E-37(2), *ibid.*; Bayne-Jones to Whitney, October 14, 1949, in Folder 4, Box 2, Secretary Treasurer Papers, 1911–1960, MANY; materials in Folders 6 and 7, Box 2, Secretary Treasurer, Society of the New York Hospital, Papers (Runyon), 1927–1978, MANY. Also of interest are the Minutes of the Executive Committee of the Board of Governors of New York Hospital, November 9, 1948, pp. 129–30, MANY.

reputation he had gained caused the American College of Physicians to present him its medal in preventive medicine, B-J chose to speak on "The Hospital as a Center of Preventive Medicine." His audience at the Waldorf-Astoria comprised four thousand specialists in internal medicine, and his paper became one of his most popular and influential. He urged that hospitals' outpatient services be viewed as a means to prevent, as well as to cure, illness. He wished to see diagnostic clinics expanded with the aim of forestalling illness. He suggested that consultation services for both doctors and patients in the community be enlarged. He favored the growth of group practice both inside and outside the hospital, and he urged the development of home-care programs based in the hospital. He wanted education and training in preventive medicine and, of course, more research in the field. Perhaps idealistically, he hoped to combine personal attention to the patient with institutional growth and social medicine.[24]

The response was immediate and heartening—"more than anything of the kind that ever happened to me before," said B-J. At Memorial-Sloan-Kettering, copies were distributed to the trustees and the board. A Philadelphia physician summed up his own reading of the paper: "The point of view needs to be changed from that of curative to that of preventive and prophylactic medicine. . . . Health rather than sickness should be stressed." A Sloan-Kettering expert called it a "classic document," unique in that it recommended precise steps and therefore formed a basis for institutional policy.[25] Certainly B-J had hit a nerve; the active propagation of health was to become a theme of American society over the next generation.

Yet his essay in medical statesmanship did nothing to alter the problems of the center, of which the most intractable remained the deficit. Post-

24. Bayne-Jones, "The Hospital as a Center of Preventive Medicine," *Annals of Internal Medicine*, XXXI (July, 1949), 7–16. See also E. H. Lewinski-Corwin, *The Hospital Situation in Greater New York: Report of a Survey of Hospitalization in New York City by the Public Health Committee of the New York Academy of Medicine* (New York, 1924), 18, 310–11, 339–40.

25. Quotations, in order: Bayne-Jones to Everett S. Elwood, editor of *The Diplomate*, November 21, 1949; Edward L. Bortz to Bayne-Jones, September 8, 1949; C. P. Rhoads to Bayne-Jones, n.d., (copy), all in E-59(3), Box 27, SBJC.

war conditions reshaped the sources of philanthropy, the craft and cost of nursing, and ultimately the meaning of charity itself.

One pressure point was the funding of research. Much of the money now came from the government. The usual medical alarms of prewar days—federal control over researchers, loss of scientific freedom—had turned out to be much exaggerated. During the war even the armed services had learned the lessons that research was essential and not to be rigidly confined. The center's problems lay in the costs that abundance brought with it. Research grants never paid the entire overhead they incurred. Heat, light, cleaning, upkeep, telephone service, insurance, sickness benefits for workers, and pensions had to be paid, and all, in some degree difficult to measure, resulted from work done under federal or foundation or private grants. Yet the center depended far too much on its income from grants to turn them down.[26]

Another postwar phenomenon was a shortage of trained nurses, resulting in part from an expanded job market for women. The shortage compelled changes in hours, pay, and status. In 1948, beds and whole wards of the hospital had to be closed down for lack of nurses; the college's program was handicapped by the loss of teaching wards. B-J, in his sixth decade, had to rethink his own conventional view of the handmaidenly role of nurses. Two people assisted his effort to change: Nan was in many ways a believer in female liberation born too soon; and Eli Ginzberg, a younger friend of B-J's from the days in the surgeon general's office, was teaching at Columbia University's School of Business and doing pioneering studies of nursing and medical economics.

The foundations of the latter, Ginzberg warned in 1947, were "worm-eaten and crumbling," a sentiment with which B-J could only agree. Ginzberg's study of nursing echoed many earlier analysts who traced the salaries traditional for nurses to the low wages and poor employment opportunities of women before World War I. The conditions had changed, but the pay, relatively speaking, had not. Calling for greater cooperation among doctors and nurses and reduced medical authoritarianism, Ginzberg cited the army as his own introduction to nursing reform. In the military, the nurse had been an officer, with assistants—enlisted corpsmen, WACs, prisoners of war—to do the un-

26. JAB Minutes, September 24, 1948, p. 571, in E-36(3), and January 21, 1949, p. 601, in E-37(1), both in Box 25, SBJC.

skilled labor. She had faced the medical officers with her status enhanced, not diminished, by the uniform.

During 1948, B-J joined a committee headed by Ginzberg to survey the status of nursing on behalf of Columbia Teachers' College. The
committee's report called for the systematic professionalization of nursing. Underlining the military analogy, it proposed a small group of
highly qualified professionals at the top of the profession and a larger
group of practical nurses to handle the housekeeping, clerical, and non-
technical duties of patient care. In taking this line, the committee invaded an area long debated by nurses themselves, uncertain whether
aides and attendants (and, since the 1930s, licensed practical nurses)
enhanced their status or threatened their jobs.

But the shift from a depression-era surplus of nurses to a wartime and postwar shortage made inevitable the changes that Ginzberg
sought to legitimate and organize by appealing to the military model.
In fact, change was already coming to the center. In August, 1947, registered nurses were relieved of many lowly tasks. In 1949 the New York
State Nurse Practice Act went into effect, prohibiting the unlicensed
from nursing but allowing them to carry out subsidiary tasks.[27]

In addition to research and nursing costs, the cost of treating non-
paying patients rose constantly, provoking bitter quarrels between hospital and college. By 1957 the deficit stood at $690,000, exclusive of
depreciation, and the greatest losses were in the free wards and the
outpatient department—precisely the areas that were most important
for clinical teaching. The result was a sharp attack by the hospital's governors on the costs of teaching; a demand that Cornell assume more of
the burden; and—by implication, though the meaning was clear—a
scathing critique of B-J's financial stewardship. The Society of the New
York Hospital asked the board to make recommendations for reducing
the deficit "in relation to teaching, training and research" by $200,000
to $300,000.

The board duly gave the job to B-J, who had no choice but to

27. Materials in E-65, Box 27, SBJC; Ginzberg quotation in New York *Herald Tribune*, November 21, 1948. On the situation in nursing, see Susan M. Reverby, *Ordered to
Care: The Dilemma of American Nursing, 1850–1945* (Cambridge, Mass., 1987), 193–96,
and Barbara Melosh, *"The Physician's Hand" : Work Culture and Conflict in American Nursing* (Philadelphia, 1982), 178–83.

become the agent of changes he found distasteful, notably the conversion of ward space to semiprivate rooms. Hospital physicians disliked the idea as much as B-J and the college did; everyone knew that the change would make the hospital less serviceable to the poor, impede research, and impair the development of clinical specialties. Before the Joint Administrative Board, debate was extended and unhappy. B-J, admitting that it was "not entirely a good thing to do" and "a forced expedient," expressed the hope that soon everyone would be covered either by government or by private insurance plans.[28]

In the end even the dissenters went along. The hospital was changing under pressure of the deficit, and nobody could halt the process. The institution's shield showed the Good Samaritan and bore the words of Jesus, "Go thou and do likewise." The age of Blue Cross and a hundred other hospital plans—and of Medicare to follow—gave an entirely new meaning to the old command. What seemed to be ending was charity itself, in the old sense, and conformity to the new way was not to be avoided.[29]

Though his places of work were the office and the boardroom, B-J also addressed himself on many occasions to the students. The young men and women in white lab coats or hospital green were the real issue in the quarrels over ward beds, cost sharing, the relation with Sloan-Kettering, and half a dozen other matters. They gave the center much of its life and all of its future. In his years there B-J seemed drawn to the students as never before; curious about them, as an aging man is about the young; alarmed for them, and for the trend of the times they must live in.

The events of the late forties and early fifties—the spread of

28. JAB Minutes, May 18, 1951, p. 782, in E-37(5), Box 26, SBJC. See also Report of a Committee on the Financial Problems of The New York Hospital, to John Hay Whitney, June 3, 1950; Bayne-Jones, Notes on the Committee, January 26, 1950; Report and Recommendations in Relation to Reduction of the Deficit of The New York Hospital, October 30, 1951, p. 1, all in Folder 3, Box 2, President's Papers, 1945–1975, MANY.

29. Bayne-Jones, Report and Recommendations Relative to Reduction of the Deficit of The New York Hospital, October 30, 1951, p. 3, in Folder 3, Box 2, President's Papers, 1945–1975; MANY; JAB Minutes, September 21, 1951, pp. 790–91, and October 24, 1951, p. 805, both in E-37(7), Box 26, SBJC.

atomic weapons, the onset of the Cold War, the outbreak of fighting in Korea, and the rise of McCarthyism—troubled him deeply and compelled response. He tried to pass his concerns on to the young, telling one graduating class that he was amazed at the "terrorism in the country" that could make a man fail to stand by friends accused of subversion. But he understood, too, that the students were part of the problem. Commentators of the time noted the peculiar listless passivity of young people; B-J viewed it with astonishment. Lacking the experience of the veterans who had preceded them, students tended to accept what they were told, growing into balanced, quizzical men and women marked by a reluctance to commit themselves, a lack of normal rebelliousness, and a superficial maturity. B-J warned them that the "apathy of acceptance" helped to make intellectual terrorism possible, and called for a revival of the nerve and optimism without which a doctor could not hope to foster health, prevent disease, or cure it.[30]

In speaking to a new class at the medical college—a paper later printed and much praised—he abandoned the academic habit of lining up authorities and relied upon his own intuitive sense of what the medical art was about. Ultimately, he argued, medicine depends upon the "biological initiative," a self-sustaining natural process beyond human control. Medicine's task is to liberate that process, giving "scope to the biological initiative of man" by preventing disabilities and conserving human resources. Hence medicine by its nature had always been an agency for the objective study and understanding of human behavior, "a social science even before social sciences were differentiated." As such, despite its cults and fads, it had freed humanity from enslaving errors, while demanding firmness and self-sacrifice from those who practiced it. No one could be a good physician without being a free man. But what was freedom?

For his surprising coda, he turned as far as he could from the authoritarianism that oppressed the world: to another physician, François Rabelais, and to his call for an ultimate liberation. "I wish," said B-J, "there were above our doors the old motto, 'Do As You Wish,'" for "'men that are free, of gentle birth, well-bred, and at home in civilized company possess a natural instinct that inclines them to virtue and

30. Bayne-Jones, Notes for an Address to the Graduating Class, June 11, 1952, in E-52 (Commencement), Box 27, SBJC; reported in New York *Times*, June 12, 1952.

saves them from vice. This instinct they call their honor.'" If B-J had a matured philosophy, this was it—a highly personal compound of science and honor, skepticism and ideal vision. He believed that a state of being was real, and possible for humankind, in which generous and compassionate behavior becomes the norm of the spirit that respects itself and despises compulsion.[31]

In the age of Cold War and frozen certitudes, he tried to convey to his young people optimism, fearlessness, and trust in the wayward creativity of life. "I would take the Ode to the West Wind to heart and repeat [it]," he told one graduating class, "if we were not all so sophisticated and shy." They lived in the winter of history. Could spring be far behind? A childless man, seeing his own days shorten, he hoped to bequeath them a life of usefulness and honor, "lasting until you yourselves pass on the healing power of the good physician to your own successors."[32]

B-J liked to say that he retired often because each time brought him a banquet. As he prepared to leave the medical center in June, 1953, John Hay Whitney held an "enormous feast" at the Links Club in his honor. Guests included the board of governors, the Cornell trustees, members of the faculty, and prominent New Yorkers like Francis Cardinal Spellman. Friends and former antagonists alike praised B-J's accomplishments and noted that he had "endeared himself to us all in the midst of difficult negotiations."[33] Nobody mentioned the deficit, which had begun to climb again. And in fact B-J, looking back on his tenure, would later conclude that despite his efforts he had lost the combat with the numbers while winning other and less tangible victories. He left a united and growing center, better integrated than ever before, and he had re-created a position of leadership that continued after him.

31. Bayne-Jones, "Freedom Inherent in Medicine and Physicians," *The Diplomates,* XXIII (March, 1951), 93–96. The internal quotation is from the conclusion to *Gargantua.*

32. Bayne-Jones, Notes for an Address to the Graduating Class, June 11, 1952, in E-52, Box 27, SBJC.

33. David P. Barr, address, [June 11, 1953], in E-50(2), Box 26, SBJC. See also Whitney to Bayne-Jones, May 12, 1953, Lucille Wright, Secretary of the Nursing Faculty, to Bayne-Jones, June 29, 1953, *ibid.* Following a lengthy tenure by Hinsey, the chief administrative officer's position was allowed to lapse again.

With that he had to be content, as he turned south to a new role in Washington, where increasingly the critical decisions on national medical policy were being made. B-J was to have a part in those decisions, for he had been summoned to direct the army's program of medical research and soon would play leading roles in the Public Health Service as well.[34]

34. Phillips interview, 987.

TEN

Statesman of Medicine

Ambitious people often find a final destination in Washington, and by no means an uncomfortable one. The city on the Potomac has traditionally been both capital and village, a political powerhouse that has somehow kept a bit of amiable provincialism as well. Here B-J and Nan returned in the early summer of 1953, after seven years' absence. Neither would leave Washington for long again.

The city was especially right for B-J. To have reached at last the center of centers, to live in a middle-sized, half-southern city, to do congenial work, to associate with top dogs who accepted him as an equal—how could he ask for more? He found in Washington a compound of his roots and his ambitions, a good place to live and, across the river in Arlington, a place to rest.

For a month the Bayne-Joneses stayed at the Dolly Madison house on Wisconsin Avenue, a dignified 150-year-old dwelling owned by a friend. Then, after several attempts, they found their permanent dwelling in a house that stood just west of Sheridan Circle. Nan worked over her house with loving care; a visitor saw her at the kitchen sink, scrubbing layers of paint from old brasswork. She and B-J divided the place between them: her bedroom and his study on the second floor, his bedroom and her sewing room on the third. So, as perhaps they had always wanted to, they lived alone in each other's company.

In Washington the job makes the man, and B-J's position, added to old contacts, assured a widening circle of acquaintances. He and Nan were most at home among the scientists, the soldiers and government savants, the judges and upper-level bureaucrats who sustained the political merry-go-round without joining it. But they also knew a few of the politically powerful. Dean Acheson, lately secretary of state, was an old friend and occasional enemy from the Yale Corporation. Through Acheson, B-J developed a lively friendship with Supreme Court Justice Felix Frankfurter, that "small, noisy man," as *Newsweek* called him, brilliant liberal intellectual and inveterate gossip, to whom "talk was . . . ambrosia." The three were together in Frankfurter's apartment on the afternoon of October 18, 1962, when Acheson's troubled face and burdened manner gave B-J his first inkling of the onset of the Cuban missile crisis.[1]

Baltimore, Nan's hometown and B-J's long-time residence, was only forty miles away, and he was quick to renew acquaintance with Johns Hopkins friends. His onetime students wrote him, signing half-forgotten campus nicknames and bragging a bit about their achievements in medicine. B-J pursued hobbyistic interests in a score of subjects—the medical use of lasers, paleopathology, leprosy research, the philosophy of science—and showed himself a practiced after-dinner speaker, able to talk well about what he understood and almost as well about what he did not. He belonged to several clubs, the Cosmos, the Metropolitan, and the Army and Navy. He had always been a clubbable man, and Washington delighted in such institutions. He settled into his new life, aware from the beginning, perhaps, that his nomadic days were over.[2]

But for all its charm, the city like the nation had been vastly transformed by the Korean War, then nearing its end. On July 27, the fighting on the battered Asian peninsula came to an end. All along the bloody summits that ran from the Imjin River to the Sea of Japan—T-Bone Hill, Pork Chop Hill, Old Baldy, White Horse Mountain, Jane Russell Hill, Heartbreak Ridge, Luke the Gook's Castle—"wild cheers broke out from American GI's" as the thunderous barrages that shook the last day stopped suddenly at 10 P.M., and the war ended, as it had begun, in darkness. The fighting left many mementoes: to the White House, the Republican administration of Dwight D. Eisenhower; to the world, the Cold War in its most intense form; and to Washington, the foundations of the national security state.[3]

As technical director of research and development for the surgeon general of the army, B-J's duties were familiar ones. The government's com-

1. Acheson ceased to be secretary of state in 1953 but as an elder statesman·was summoned by the Kennedy Administration to give advice. See Bayne-Jones to Acheson, December 7, 1962, in I-1, Box 43, SBJC. Apparently, Bayne-Jones and Nan moved into the house on Massachusetts Avenue in August, 1958. On Frankfurter, see *Newsweek*, March 8, 1965, p. 30.

2. See materials in I-1, SBJC, and Bayne-Jones's Biographical Notes, in Folder 3, Secretary Treasurer's Records, Society of the New York Hospital, MANY.

3. Washington *Evening Star*, July 27, 1953.

mitment to research continued to expand, as it had with few interruptions since World War II. His Research and Development Division contained branches devoted to medical, surgical, and psychological research, and it controlled the funds of what had become, in an era of service unification, the Armed Forces Epidemiological Board.

B-J reviewed proposals for research projects, judged their scientific value and the competence of the proponents, evaluated the results of their work, and kept his military chief and the surgeon general abreast of the program. He dealt with the medical departments of the other armed services, each of which had its own research arm. Relations with the National Research Council (NRC) were close; B-J did much to shape the organization and activities of its division of medical research, and in turn NRC experts helped to formulate the Army's total research program.[4]

Everywhere he found old acquaintances. But two wars and the research boom they brought had greatly expanded the old-boy network's membership and power. An elective elite, clubby, contentious, increasingly open to Jews and other onetime outsiders, B-J's arm of the Establishment gathered in the Society of Medical Consultants of the Armed Forces—a virtual who's who of influential doctors with a soft spot for the military. The roster included the surgeon generals of the army and the Public Health Service, Michael E. DeBakey, William C. Menninger, and Paul R. Hawley—once the European Theater's chief surgeon and more recently the president of the American College of Surgeons. Eli Ginzberg was a member, as were several wheelhorses of the Army Surgeon General's office, including his senior consultant Isidor A. Ravdin.[5]

4. Bayne-Jones, Memorandum for Col. R. L. Hullinghorst, MC, Chief, Research and Development Division, subject: Advisory Services, December 18, 1956, in G-3(1), Box 33, SBJC; Phillips interview, 985–90. In the usual confusing manner of Washington organizations, the organization for which Bayne-Jones worked began as the Research and Development Board, later became the Research and Development Division, and still later the Research and Development Command. These changes are not noted in the text; they did, however, mark the increasing importance of research to the surgeon general.

5. See materials in G-2(1), Box 32, SBJC, especially Committee on Preventive Medicine, Society of United States Medical Consultants: Minutes of First Meeting, March 26, 1952; and materials in G-2(3), especially Silas B. Hays, "The Society of Medical Consultants to the Armed Forces," photocopied MS, n.d.; and the roster in G-2(4), Box 33, SBJC. The society continues to exist today as a tri-service organization.

In 1954 B-J also joined the Army Scientific Advisory Panel (ASAP). The nation's potential enemies possessed superior manpower, and the American army was shrinking in the post–Korean War drawdown. Therefore, in the view of Chief of Staff Gen. Matthew B. Ridgway, the American soldier must have technological superiority that could only be sustained through research. Representatives of the Bell Telephone Laboratories, Purdue University, the New England Power System, General Electric, and other captains of industry and erudition met semiannually with representatives of the army's technical services to view sham battles, receive frank briefings, and attend banquets in the company of glittering brass. In return, they offered candid criticisms and suggested solutions to current problems of research and production. The group was a paradigm of what President Dwight D. Eisenhower had not yet named the military-industrial complex.[6]

By comparison with the army's vast concerns, the research program of the surgeon general was small potatoes. Yet in 1953, 115 universities and civilian hospitals signed 385 contracts let by B-J's division and received about half of its $10.5-million budget. This was the "extramural" program. The division also worked closely with the army's own research institutions at Walter Reed, Fort Knox's Army Medical Research Laboratory, and more specialized centers at Brooke Army Medical Center in San Antonio and at Fitzsimons Army Hospital near Denver. About $4 million went to the "in-house" program.

As he had in the past, B-J struggled to loosen the bonds of research. He sought to write contracts that specified the field of study—for example, a particular vaccine—while "allowing the investigator to follow his leads, so long as he keeps within a certain field." He liked to cite the work of his friend David Nachmansohn, a biochemist whose interest in neurotransmitters led him to long and fruitful work for the army on antidotes for the nerve gases. Such occasions delighted B-J, when pure research undertaken for love of the subject suddenly acquired urgent practical value. As an administrator, he took craftsmanlike pride in Nachmansohn's contract, which named as the end product

6. Memorandum, Ridgway to Surgeon General, May 20, 1954, subject: Reorganization of the Army Scientific Advisory Panel, in G-13, Box 34, SBJC; Hays to C/S, May 27, 1954, same subject, *ibid.*; Secretary of the Army Robert T. Stevens to Bayne-Jones, October 6, 1954, *ibid.*

discovery of "the nature of the nerve impulse," a near-metaphysical goal that liberated the scientist to follow his own path.[7]

Yet two wars had wrought vast changes in the scope of medical knowledge. Malaria appeared to be a problem largely solved by the new synthetic antimalarial primaquine. The old military curse of VD no longer seemed to matter much, because of antibiotic therapy. Many other once-deadly infections had become insignificant for similar reasons. In Korea, arterial repair carried out in the mobile surgical hospitals (MASHs) had drastically reduced the number of amputations necessary among casualties with vascular damage. Impressive advances had been made in burn treatment, in the understanding and prevention of cold injury, and in the battlefield management of injuries to the brain and spinal cord.

What was left to do? B-J asked his colleagues, probably without conscious irony. Treatment of burns in mass-casualty situations—he was, of course, thinking of nuclear warfare—needed "most serious consideration." What of stress? "The word itself is producing stress." It was time to consider seriously a concept that, as yet, was only a catchword. Military machines had to be adapted to the human beings who used them. Climatic studies were a continuing necessity for forces that might have to live and fight anywhere on earth. Despite an age of medical optimism, B-J saw plenty of work to be done in developing answers to the ills resulting from the supremely stressful event of war.[8]

In looking for new and promising lines of research, B-J's old interest in nutrition revived. During the Korean War, a top-secret army study showed that South Korean soldiers had often been so poorly fed by their government that their battlefield performance was impaired. As a result, nutrition studies among the nation's poorer allies had multiplied. B-J appealed for help to the Department of Defense, which found substantial sums to carry the program forward. Then an interdepartmental committee was formed that brought together the armed services, the Public Health Service, the departments of State and Agricul-

7. On Nachmansohn, see Phillips interview, 1009. See also Bayne-Jones, Trends in Armed Forces Research, transcript of speech at annual meeting of Society of Medical Consultants to the Armed Forces, Walter Reed Army Medical Center, November 23, 1953, p. 8, in G-2(3), Box 32, SBJC.

8. Bayne-Jones, Trends, 14; Phillips interview, 100.

ture, and the National Research Council. Studies grew to include the civil populations of friendly countries from whom the troops were drawn. Financed at first by the military and then by the Agency for International Development with assistance from the National Institutes of Health, the program gave B-J great satisfaction, "an instance of how a great thing can grow from a very small little acorn." In a way, it was his Institute of Nutrition, achieved at last on a worldwide basis.[9]

B-J's agenda for military medical research also included the study of psychochemicals—substances intended to disorient or disable enemy soldiers instead of killing or doing permanent injury to them. ("Very wise and promising," he noted.) In time, the combat use of nonlethal chemicals foundered on several problems, notably the impossibility of controlling concentrations under field conditions. But B-J's interest showed that he was ready to use medical research to develop new weapons as well as new techniques of prevention and treatment. In this respect he followed the changing outlook of the surgeon general of the army, who committed himself in the mid-fifties to increased research into biological warfare (BW).[10]

B-J reentered the field through several doors. One was the Armed Forces Epidemiological Board (AFEB), whose work the Research and Development Division funded. In 1955 the board noted that the surgeon general was exploring the possibility of an enhanced role and moved to become his chief adviser on BW. An agreement signed on February 3, 1956, with the chief chemical officer took the Medical Service beyond its traditional work in providing defense against enemy biological attacks and into a shared responsibility for all army research in the field. A member of B-J's division provided liaison and described the new arrangement to the AFEB: The chemical corps would seek money for BW research from Congress, with the surgeon general's help if needed; research money would then be funneled through the Research and Development Division to the AFEB, which would let

9. On the nutrition program, see Phillips interview, 996–99; Albert E. Cowdrey, *The Medics' War: U.S. Army in the Korean War* (Washington, 1987), 332–33.

10. Revised Project Officer List, August 1, 1956, Research and Development Division, Office of the Surgeon General, Department of the Army, in G-3(1), Box 33, SBJC; Bayne-Jones, [Notes on] Walter Reed Army Institute of Research, February 12–13, 1959, in G-3(4), Box 33, *ibid.*

the necessary contracts. B-J's old Commission on Epidemiological Survey had been abolished but now was resuscitated to handle the BW contracts.[11]

By the time B-J himself rejoined the AFEB in 1958, work on BW had become routine. The surgeon general of the army spent about $1 million a year on BW during 1958, 1959, and 1960. Some $875,000 went to the U.S. Army Medical Unit at Camp Detrick and the Walter Reed Army Institute of Research in Washington, while the remainder was parceled out to contractors, including the University of Maryland, Ohio State University, and Peter Bent Brigham Hospital in Boston. Work included experiments with a Russian vaccine for respiratory tularemia; human volunteers were immunized, then "challenged" with suspensions of *Pasteurella tularensis* in aerosols. Experiments with Rift Valley fever and Venezuelan equine encephalomyelitis vaccines were also under way by 1959. The commission worked on production in vitro of anthrax toxin; sought to determine "effective and lethal doses" of staphylococcal enterotoxin for experimental animals; and carried out human trials to establish the infectivity of typhoid. Its other endeavors were secret.[12]

In 1959 the AFEB made an effort to consolidate all medical research in biological warfare under itself. Members recognized the necessity, if they did so, of abandoning the old claim that they provided research only into defensive aspects of BW, but as they pointed out, that would involve little practical change. Even the development of a vaccine had offensive implications, because friendly forces would have to be immunized before any disease could be used against an enemy. "The Board now recognizes that offensive and defensive aspects are inseparable. Diplomatically, the defensive aspects can be stressed as in

11. See materials in Minutes of the First Annual Meeting, AFEB, September 19–20, 1949, Box 1, and Minutes of the Special Meeting of the AFEB, February 6, 1956, Box 4, in AFEB Meeting Files, RG 334, NARA.

12. Minutes of the Executive Session, AFEB, in Box 5, AFEB Meeting Files. See also December, 1959, Report of the Director of the Commission on Epidemiological Survey to the AFEB, in Box 9, AFEB Meeting Files; T. E. Woodward and W. D. Tigertt, "Review of the Activities of the Commission on Epidemiological Survey," *Military Medicine*, CXXVI (1961), 37–39. Tigertt commanded the U.S. Army Medical Unit at Fort Detrick, and Woodward, a Typhus Commission alumnus, headed the Department of Medicine at the University of Maryland School of Medicine.

the past, since there is a need to know all about the offensive aspects in order to develop proper defensive capabilities against BW and CW."[13]

Did this declaration measure some fundamental change in thinking brought about by the wars? Or did it merely signal a gain in candor? In either case, the board's ambitions were not fulfilled; bureaucratic confusion worsened, and BW remained the plaything of many competing agencies. Yet the surgeon general remained deeply involved. B-J had helped to launch the whole BW program in the early days of World War II, and he served without apparent question the new commitment of the Medical Service. The weapons of BW were no more appalling than many others and were far less likely to be used than either chemical or nuclear weapons. Nevertheless, his contribution to their development was a curious turn in the career of a physician long devoted to preventive medicine and formed the dark side of his Washington career under the national security state that had emerged from the Korean War.[14]

Despite his ties to the Epidemiological Board—which continued until 1965—his career took a marked civilian turn from the mid-fifties onward. He retired in 1956 from his post as technical director of research for the Medical Service. To a friend he explained, "I decided I had best move out when I am well and before my D day (Disintegration day) came around."[15]

But in fact he had no intention of abandoning his career at the age of sixty-seven. As usual, B-J found no trouble in discerning the center of things. To a doctor that meant the Department of Health, Education and Welfare, created under the Eisenhower administration as the newest superagency, a kind of national philanthropic Pentagon. By the time he bade the board farewell, B-J was deeply involved in work with the surgeon general of the Public Health Service.

13. Minutes of the Executive Session, AFEB, May 20, 1959, p. 3, in Box 8, AFEB Meeting Files.

14. Minutes of the Executive Session of the AFEB, May 17, 1960, in Box 9, AFEB Meeting Files.

15. Bayne-Jones to Pearl L. Kendrick, University of Michigan School of Public Health, August 2, 1956, in G-13, Box 34, SBJC. On his retirement, Bayne-Jones received the army's highest civilian honor, the Decoration for Exceptional Civilian Service. See the Washington Star, July 1, 1956.

A year after his valedictory to the Research and Development Division, B-J became chairman of an advisory committee established by Marion Folsom, secretary of health, education and welfare, to review the programs and policies of the National Institutes of Health (NIH) and their impacts on medical education and research. Revolutionary changes were under way at the NIH. The institutes now formed a complex of laboratories at Bethesda, Maryland, on Washington's northwestern perimeter. During the Eisenhower years a powerful coalition emerged in Congress, devoted to improving the nation's health with federal money. Politicians both liberal and conservative discovered the advantages of being perceived by their constituents as battlers against deadly diseases. James A. Shannon, a physician who had done research for the Army Epidemiological Board during World War II, was appointed director of the NIH in 1955. He presided over a golden age of expansion, during which federal funding rose from $98 million to $1.4 billion a year.[16]

When Congress doubled his budget in 1957, Shannon asked for an advisory group to set forth the principles that should govern the operation of NIH. "And I suggested," he later recalled, "that the best person to head that group was Bayne-Jones . . . and [Folsom] called Bayne-Jones down and Bayne-Jones in a year did a superb job and set forth a set of principles that I found totally acceptable to me, but more important they [were] totally acceptable to the Secretary."[17]

B-J's committee held its first meeting in the secretary's office on October 10. Its members were not quite an assembly of his cronies, but all were well known to him, a cross-section of his world and of the groups that were interested in medical research and education. Of the ten members, five were present or former academics and the others represented great chemical and drug firms. After Folsom gave his

16. Bayne-Jones to Maxwell E. Lapham, July 9, 1957, in Folder 8, Box 1, SBJT; Phillips interview, 1051–53; Victoria A. Harden, *Inventing the NIH: Federal Biomedical Research Policy, 1887–1934* (Baltimore, 1986), 184–85; Patterson, *Dread Disease*, 182–83. On the growth in NIH appropriations (and the more informative growth in constant dollars), see James B. Wyngaarden, "The National Institutes of Health in Its Centennial Year," *Science*, CCXXXVIII (August 21, 1987), 869–74.

17. Interview with James Shannon, January 11, 1984, pp. 29–30 of transcript, at NLM; see also James Shannon, "The National Institutes of Health: Some Critical Years, 1955–1957," *Science*, CCXXXVIII (August 21, 1987), 865–68.

charge to the consultants, and B-J made the requisite promise of "best effort, hard work and devotion," Shannon briefly described his rapidly expanding empire. He pointed out that research and development in all fields absorbed a rising proportion of the gross national product, and that medical research was keeping pace with the trend. The NIH supported research, the training of researchers, and the construction of facilities for research. How and when to broaden the three areas of support "constitutes the core of the policy problem" at NIH, Shannon declared.[18]

A busy year followed, as B-J led the effort to draw up a rational blueprint for NIH's future. Throughout, he found himself retracing his earlier steps as a medical administrator and policymaker. One of his panel's first actions was to endorse unanimously full federal assumption of the indirect costs of research that had plagued B-J in New York. More basic was the question of what the federal support of research did to the universities that accepted it.

The problem was that NIH had its single mission—basic research—but that of the medical schools was more complex: to teach, to research, and to conserve knowledge as well. As Shannon himself said, no funds were available to enable the universities to maintain their balance, and hence to keep their fundamental character. Yet the country needed practicing physicians; sophisticated knowledge meant nothing unless it was applied, and research was ultimately pointless if it degraded training. The question went deep, and the consultants were divided not so much among themselves as within their own minds. Well aware of the problems created by the golden shower that had descended on the laboratories, they remained deeply committed to the ultimate good of expanding medical knowledge. B-J was at any rate clear-sighted: federal control had in fact come to medical schools, not by the much-feared avenue of compulsion, but by "allurement and seduction." But no more than the others could he see a way to release medical education from the golden vise, except to spend more federal money on teaching and construction as well.[19]

18. Minutes of the First Meeting, Consultants on Medical Education and Research, Office of the Secretary, Department of Health, Education and Welfare, October 10, 1957, pp. 1, 5–21. See also Phillips interview, 1054–55.

19. Minutes of 3rd Consultants' Meeting, December 16–17, 1957, pp. 2–3, 20–23, in G-33(3), Box 36, SBJC; Phillips interview, 1067.

Many of the committee's conclusions were soothing: that the NIH in general had done an excellent job; that its grant program had contrived to avoid bureaucratic lassitude as well as bureaucratic interference with science. As for the money question, there was really no alternative to federal funding in steadily increasing quantities. Growth controlled by caution was the answer. As against the congressional juggernaut, B-J's committee favored continued steady growth in federal spending to $500 million a year by 1970, or one-half the estimated total of all expenditure, public and private, on medical research. The needs of education would be met by "large federal appropriations" to assist the construction and staffing of fourteen to twenty new medical schools, to assure that the ratio of physicians to population did not fall.

In effect, said *Time,* the committee favored "no blitz, but a powerhouse drive down the field." No wonder that it pleased the secretary; as Shannon later said, its main function was to "place a stamp of high approval" on the pre-existing aims of the NIH.[20]

Recommending more of the same, especially more money, rarely makes enemies. In sharp contrast was B-J's final effort for the Public Health Service. He undertook wittingly to hurt major interests and anger substantial parts of the public by recommending governmental interference with a great national industry and a cherished, though lethal, habit.

Since his days at Yale with the Childs fund B-J had never quite lost touch with cancer research, if only because so many of his friends continued to die of the disease. Shortly after he came to Washington, he became involved in the final illness of one of the city's most powerful men, the longtime senator from Ohio and perennial contender for the Republican presidential nomination, Robert A. Taft.

B-J had known this unusual man since 1909 when, as a Yale student, he had shared the Taft family's first Christmas in the White House. He and Robert Taft became friends, and later participants in the secret rites of Skull and Bones. Beginning in 1937, Taft served for

20. *Times,* July 21, 1958, pp. 34–35; Department of Health, Education, and Welfare, *The Advancement of Medical Research and Education Through the Department of Health, Education, and Welfare* (Washington, 1958), especially 1–11, 60.

years on the Yale Corporation; he and his wife, Martha, accepted the Bayne-Joneses' hospitality at New Haven and invited them in turn to visit the senator's "Sears-Roebuck house" in Washington. Taft helped B-J get appropriations for the Epidemiological Board; B-J contributed to Taft's last senate race, while privately hoping that his admired friend, whose quirky independence sometimes declined into mere crankiness, might *not* become president.[21]

When Taft in 1953 fell ill at a critical moment in public affairs—the new Republican Congress was in session, the Russian dictator Josef Stalin had just died, and the Eisenhower administration was hinting at the possibility of nuclear war in order to force the People's Republic of China to make peace in Korea—B-J was one of the first outside the senator's family to know that the trouble was cancer. Taft was determined to keep his illness secret. How, then, was he to have treatment? B-J, as friend, physician, and man of affairs, had to find a way.

His first scheme turned out badly. He checked Taft into New York Hospital as "Howard Roberts." Memorial Hospital was too revealing, but its proximity and the fact that the Medical Center, Memorial, and Sloan-Kettering were affiliated under agreements that B-J had helped to engineer meant that some of the best talent in the country would be available. It was a perfect scheme, flawed only in that the secret could not possibly be kept. Within twenty-four hours the New York *Daily News* reported both Taft's hospitalization and his pseudonym, from which the senator's colleagues drew the obvious and correct conclusion. Thereafter B-J made no more errors, as he counseled the family and the medical staff through the remainder of the ordeal. Taft died on July 31 at Memorial; on autopsy, pathologists found the origin of the cancer in one of his lungs.[22]

B-J's penultimate service was to help the family go public with the facts of the case. On the evening of July 31 he contacted Alfred Friendly, editor of the Washington *Post*, while Taft's physician spoke to

21. Taft to Bayne-Jones, April 10, 1941, in I-28(1), Box 45, SBJC. In Phillips interview, 507, Bayne-Jones confesses, "I would not have wanted to see [Taft] be president."

22. Bayne-Jones, Summary of medical record of Mr. Robert A. Taft, June 6, 1953, and The New York Hospital, Summary of Findings, Taft Robert Senator, n.d., and other related materials, all in I-28(2) and I-28(3), Box 45, SBJC.

the editors of *Time*. As a result, the public received an accurate, unsensational account of the senator's illness and death—another blow to the old tradition that cancer was an unmentionable illness. His last service was to serve on a memorial committee whose carillon tower, set among pleasant trees just north of the Senate, remains Washington's only monument to a member of the upper house.[23]

The national crusade against cancer, to which B-J had contributed during the thirties, was by now in full swing. Gone were the days when, as he recalled, "many investigators knew that work on problems of cancer would break a man's heart, if not his reputation." A great expansion in cancer research had begun after V-J Day, and from 1946 through 1951 cancer research took 46 percent of the government funding, as well as 54 percent of the private funding, for medical research in the United States, aggregating $28.4 million. By 1961 the NCI's annual funding along had risen to $110 million.

Yet as basic research advanced—uncovering the secrets of cellular growth, bodily control mechanisms, the action of viruses and carcinogens—the long-sought cure or cures for cancer remained elusive. Incidence grew; lung cancer especially increased with dismaying speed; and studies multiplied that suggested a link between some forms of cancer and a pervasive habit of the twentieth century, cigarette smoking.[24]

In 1959, Surgeon General Leroy E. Burney asked B-J to become a member of the National Advisory Cancer Council (NACC), established by Congress to advise his office on cancer programs and to recommend grants for extramural research. The council's members were leaders in the fundamental sciences, the medical sciences, education,

23. Charles P. Taft to Natalie Moorman, July 15, 1953, and other related materials in I-28(3), SBJC; see also Summary of Findings, Taft; *Time*, August 10, 1953, p. 57; Jhan and June Robbins, "The Great Untold Story of Senator Taft, Eight Weeks to Live," *The Week* (magazine), New York *Herald Tribune*, January 17, 1954, pp. 8–9.

24. Patterson, *Dread Disease*, 171; Bayne-Jones, "Aspects of Cancer Research in the United States of America," 9, Bertner Foundation Lecture, Houston, April 25, 1952, in E-69(3), Box 28, SBJC. See also Stella Leche Deignan and Esther Miller, "The Support of Research in Medical and Allied Fields for the Period 1946 through 1951," *Science*, CXV (March 28, 1952), 336; Leonard A. Scheele, "A General View of Cancer Research: The Fourth James Ewing Memorial Lecture," *Bulletin of the New York Academy of Medicine*, 2nd ser., XXV (November, 1949), 671–97.

and public affairs. B-J's tenure was brief; he clashed with Shannon and resigned. This, of course, was one of the joys of the retired state, having to take no nonsense from any man, not even the head of the NIH.

Yet B-J's brief NACC period extended his connection with the Public Health Service and gave him a refresher course in recent cancer research. His skirmish with Shannon evidently did him no harm with Burney's successor as surgeon general, Luther Terry. On the contrary, when in 1962 a candidate was needed for a far more sensitive and important job, Terry turned to B-J as much perhaps for his demonstrated independence as for his expertise.[25]

For three decades, he reminded B-J, researchers had raised with ever greater insistence the possibility that smoking might cause cancer. Reports of their work had spread so widely that government action might be necessary. The first step must be an investigation of the merits of the case by a blue-ribbon panel. B-J demurred, but Terry was insistent. With reluctance B-J prepared, late in his seventy-third year, to strike a last blow at the old enemy.[26]

Medical research touched politics at few points more sensitive than the carcinogenicity of tobacco. In 1962 the U.S. Department of Agriculture reported that American growers were producing over two billion pounds of tobacco annually; that in the preceding year 520,000 farms grew the plant; that some 700,000 farm families in sixteen states derived $1.6 billion from its sale; and that tobacco ranked fourth in value among national crops, though it covered only a small percentage of the American farmland. But tobacco was more than a crop; it was an industry, and the United States led the world both in production and in sales. Cigarette companies were corporate giants; magazines, newspapers, radio, and television all battened on cigarette advertising. As to the underlying attraction that made so many people use tobacco, B-J had personal experience: until 1951, when his ulcer persuaded him to give up the habit, he had been a chain smoker.[27]

Yet since the 1930s, evidence had been accumulating that linked

25. Materials in G-39, Box 37, SBJC, especially Bayne-Jones to Terry, October 23, 1961, referring to Shannon's Memorandum, October 9, 1961.
26. Bayne-Jones to I. Ridgeway Trimble, of the Medical and Chirurgical Faculty of the State of Maryland, November 26, 1962, in I-3, Box 42, SBJC.
27. Statement on the Importance of Tobacco to American Agriculture, November 9, 1962, in H-3, Box 38, *ibid.*

tobacco to cancer. By 1954 the evidence had become so pressing that the industry founded its own research program in an attempt to counter the spreading popular distrust. By 1962, under pressure from national health groups, President John F. Kennedy was ready to back his surgeon general's desire to establish an expert advisory committee. In all probability, the White House saw an opportunity to distance itself from a troubling issue, quiet critics, and delay the necessity for establishing a national policy on smoking and health.[28]

The ten men who made up the committee—all physicians save two—were selected by Terry from a panel prepared by the Public Health Service after discussions with interested federal agencies, the volunteer health agencies, and the tobacco industry. All the members enjoyed high professional reputations, several were smokers, and none had taken a strong public position for or against smoking. B-J played a special role, one that his fellow members did not know: Terry chose him in part to be his personal representative (or perhaps mole) and to keep him informed on the committee's deliberations. B-J was also listed as special consultant to the committee staff, giving him a direct hand in the preparation of the report.[29]

Assistance for the group came from the outside—from information supplied without charge by the American Cancer Society, by the Roswell Park Memorial Institute in Buffalo, and by Liggett and Myers, the cigarette manufacturers. To this degree it was able to go beyond the published evidence and into the latest laboratory findings. In any case, evidence was the key word. As the surgeon general told committee members, they were to concern themselves only with a scientific evaluation of the effects of tobacco smoking. What might be done about it was a political question and outside their competence.[30]

28. For the succession of events leading to the committee, see the Chronology, Surgeon General's Advisory Committee on Smoking and Health, October 24, 1962, in H-1, Box 38, *ibid.*

29. Phillips interview, 1110, 1115. See also Terry to Furth, September 28, 1962, Terry to Bayne-Jones, n.d., Chronology, Surgeon General's Advisory Committee on Smoking and Health, October 24, 1962, and Members of the Surgeon General's Advisory Committee on Smoking and Health, January 4, 1963, all in H-1, Box 38, SBJC. A few years later, Fieser developed cancer of the lung.

30. Phillips interview, 1107–09.

With that, the members were left to themselves. Terry attended only two meetings and then turned over the chairmanship to an assistant surgeon general who seemed to be mainly interested in assuring the speedy production of the report. After enduring inept leadership for a time, the members struck back. The committee asked the chairman to absent himself and adopted the methods of proceeding favored by the scientists. B-J, often the choice of milder-mannered colleagues to manage confrontations, informed the chairman of what had happened, and work thereafter proceeded without him.

Deliberations moved forward with energy. By grace of what he called the committee's "declaration of independence," B-J emerged in his usual role of manager and diplomat, assisting his more technically brilliant colleagues to organize their work and compose their differences. On the quiet, he may have ensured that a well-informed surgeon general developed no suspicions of his own committee. He also helped to arrange the basic agenda, by which the committee proceeded in an orderly way from accumulating precise information on major topics to general conclusions that could be comprehended by the intelligent layman.

Subcommittees broke up the problem: one explored tobacco; another, the ways in which tobacco was consumed; a third, the effects of smoking; a fourth, the genetic factors. Two supercommittees of specialists then sought to establish the relationship of smoking to specific diseases, and the pathologic anatomy of the smoker's lungs. B-J took for himself a typically modest and tedious task, assembling the existing laws on tobacco—his way of turning his own scientific mediocrity to good account, while supporting the work of the others.[31]

Preliminary papers outlined aspects of the technical problem. Bronchogenic carcinoma was responsible for the deaths of about 5,000 women and 35,000 men each year in the United States, a rate nine times as great as that recorded thirty years before. Increased accuracy in diagnosis did not appear to explain the increase. The theory that

31. Bayne-Jones to "Spike" [Edward P. Seymour of the Yale Alumni Fund], February 7, 1964, in H-1, Box 38, SBJC. See also Summary of Decisions Reached on Conduct of Study: Staff Paper prepared under Peter V. V. Hamill, Staff Medical Coordinator, in H-2, Box 38, *ibid.*

increased cigarette smoking was responsible was alluring but full of complex problems and unresolved riddles. At least seventeen carcinogens either were present in tobacco or were formed during the combustion process. Yet bronchogenic carcinoma had not been produced in any experimental animals by exposure to smoke alone—though mice *did* develop skin cancers after exposure to the chemical components of tobacco smoke.

Among humans, nonsmokers as well as smokers developed epidermoid cancer of the lung, though in far smaller numbers. Individual differences were profound: some heavy smokers lived to advanced ages and died ultimately of causes other than cancer of the lung. Finally, epidemiologic studies showed a consistent association between cancer of the bladder and smoking cigarettes, though it was difficult to see why.[32]

There were other problems. The most consistent source of claims that smoking had a causal role in cancer was the contrast between the mortality statistics of smokers and nonsmokers: more smokers died younger. The usual assumption was that the two populations were identical except for smoking. But was this true? Smoking was a complex form of social behavior. Were smokers brought to their habit by factors of personality and social class that might, even in the absence of smoking itself, make them more likely than other people to get certain diseases? Committee members convinced by the imposing statistics, however, saw all such arguments as "goblins."[33]

While it sorted through complex issues, the committee labored in a far from restful atmosphere. A *Newsweek* reporter saw members at work in a windowless office deep in the new National Library of Medicine amid a "white mountain of paper," a clutter of paper coffee cups and, inevitably, ashtrays: one smoked a cigarette, another puffed on a

32. Walter J. Burdette, Current Status of the Relationship between the Use of Tobacco and Health, in H-7, Box 38, *ibid.*

33. "Smoking and Lung Cancer," working paper, [December, 1962]. See also Joseph Berkson, "Smoking and Cancer in the Lung," *Proceedings of the Staff Meeting of the Mayo Clinic*, XXXV (June 22, 1960), 367–85. See also W. C. Hueper, *A Quest Into the Environmental Causes of Cancer of the Lung*, Public Health Monograph No. 36 (Washington, 1955), and Carl C. Seltzer, "Morphologic Constitution and Smoking," *Journal of the American Medical Association*, CLXXXIII (February 23, 1963), 539–645.

pipe, and a third smoked a cigar. Though the members conducted their business "as if they were working on the Manhattan A-bomb project," *Newsweek* anticipated "a loud and clear indictment of smoking."[34]

Perhaps the reporter was influenced by evidence that the public had already rendered a commonsense verdict. In November, 1962, a cancer victim sued Liggett and Myers, alleging that Chesterfield cigarettes had caused his condition; a federal jury in Pittsburgh decided that cigarette smoking was a cause of lung cancer but that the company was not liable, for the patient had "assumed a risk of lung cancer in his admittedly incessant smoking." In June, 1963, a contestant in a nationally televised game called *Password* was asked for the word that people most associated with "cigarette." He blurted, "Cancer," and the audience, *Time* reported, "roared with laughter and applause."[35]

Hence the committee's report may have refined and clarified a national consensus already formed. The fundamental argument it presented was statistical—alas for B-J and his distrust of computations! But statistics had long ceased to be a matter of counting noses, and the association between cigarette smoking and cancer was much more than a matter of age-adjusted death rates. Relying upon its epidemiologist, the committee rested its conclusion on five criteria. The first was the consistency of the association between smoking and cancer, meaning that varied ways of studying it all led to the same conclusion. The second was the strength of the association, the ratio of lung cancer rates among smokers as compared to nonsmokers. The third was the specificity of the association, meaning that the presence of either variable—smoking or lung cancer—was predictive of the other. The fourth was the temporal relationship, the fact that lung cancer in smokers followed rather than preceded the onset of smoking. The fifth was the coherence of the association, meaning that nothing in the conclusion that a causal relationship existed contradicted known fact about the natural history and biology of the disease. As B-J said, such evidence, though it did not establish causation, was more than a matter of rates or percentages only.

---

34. *Newsweek*, November 18, 1963, p. 61. See also Lois Mattox Miller and James Monahan, "The Cigarette Controversy: A Storm Is Brewing," *Reader's Digest*, August 1963, pp. 91–99.

35. *Time*, June 28, 1963, p. 73. Report on verdict in New York *Times*, November 10, 1962.

The final conclusions were emphatic. "Cigarette smoking is caus-
ally related to lung cancer in men. . . . Evaluation of the evidence leads
to the judgment that cigarette smoking is a significant factor in the
causation of laryngeal cancer in the male. . . . The evidence on the
tobacco–esophageal cancer relationship supports the belief that an association exists." Furthermore, cancer was not the only pathological
effect of smoking. Cigarette smoking was the "most important of the
causes of chronic bronchitis in the United States," and was associated
with peptic ulcer and decreased birth weight in children. Finally,
smoking was habituating but not addicting; it could be stopped, even
though predisposing constitutional and hereditary factors might exist.

Terry presented the report before television cameras at a large
press conference in the auditorium of the State Department. The members of the committee were present, and B-J noted that the room was
full of reporters, observers, and visitors. When the press conference
was over, Terry took his committee to lunch at the pleasant, columned
officers' club of Fort McNair, at the end of Generals' Row, where the
tall windows overlook Washington Channel and Potomac Park. Surely
they deserved to relax; their work had been long and hard, and the
result, as *Newsweek* called it, "monumental."

Reaction was quick. The World Health Organization demanded
action; the American Cancer Society, hitherto undecided, called for the
reduction of cigarette smoking. By asserting that cigarette smoking
killed and that it could be stopped, the committee had put maximum
pressure on the government to restrain the habit. Within a week the
Federal Trade Commission proposed warning labels for cigarette packs
and advertising; and Congress, in the face of foot-dragging by the AMA
and well-funded lobbying by tobacco interests, at last approved a
watered-down version of the warning in 1965. Cigarette advertising on
radio and television was banned in 1970. Cigarette sales fell off, rose
again, and then, in 1976, began a protracted decline. In 1984 the results
appeared as the "incidence of lung cancer among white men in America
decreased for the first time in at least fifty years."

Clearly, these developments were parts of a complex process in
which the report of the surgeon general's committee on smoking and
health was but a single landmark. Yet it did represent a major event in
the slow development of a national policy against smoking. Created to
deflect growing public criticism, the committee's decisive conclusions

WAR AND HEALING

served instead to reinforce the demand for action. For that result, B-J never attempted to take sole credit, but his influence on the outcome was great. Since the time of the Typhus Commission, he had made no more important contribution to preventive medicine.[36]

36. *Smoking and Health: Report of the Advisory Committee to the Surgeon General of the Public Health Service* (Washington, [1964]), 37, 38; *Newsweek*, January 27, 1964, p. 54. See also Patterson, *Dread Disease*, 227; Phillips interview, 1119–1120, 1129.

ELEVEN

The Past Revisited

During all the complications of his Washington career, B-J remained a man of roots as well as ambitions. The traditions he valued were embodied in personal memory, in historical scholarship, and in his family.

As ever, his clan continued to mean much to him. His nephew, Tom Denegre, a naval officer stationed in Washington, and Tom's wife, Louise, became close friends rather than youthful relations. Louise learned to know and love Nan, and—inevitably, as all people gifted with humor did—to find her solemnity an occasional source of merriment.

One troublesome member of the family passed away—Uncle Charlie Jones, whose schemes for mining coal in Virginia had begun the downfall of Stanhope Jones. Charlie died in April, 1953, at the age of eighty-seven, having survived his brother by fifty-nine years. He left an estate that proved to consist of two mining claims of "very dubious value," and his nephew Joseph Merrick Jones, a successful lawyer in New Orleans, paid for his funeral.[1]

Soon this new Joseph Jones also began to influence B-J's life. Hamilton Jones's son had grown into a "strong-minded, serious, slow-speaking, impressive man," said B-J, with an "element of command" in his character that suited his bulky, solid frame. Married well, intensively civic-minded, rising rapidly in influence and wealth, Jones was a dynamic new force in the somewhat airless world of New Orleans' merchant princes.

He served also as head of Tulane University's board of administrators, and in this capacity confronted serious problems at the medical school. Viewing B-J as a cousin—their fathers had been half-brothers—Jones saw in him a potential ally. His plea for assistance was tactful but pressing. In November, 1953, B-J told a friend that he had been elected to membership on the Board of Visitors of Tulane University, an orga-

---

1. Telegram, Joseph Merrick Jones to Bayne-Jones, April 27, 1953, in Folder 6, Box 1, SBJT.

nization that Jones had set up to bring fresh blood into the university's near-hereditary leadership.[2]

From his new advisers Jones sought help with the array of difficulties that beset the university—lack of money, a dissatisfied faculty, a university president widely perceived as ineffectual, and an antiquated physical plant. Tulane could not peacefully enjoy its traditional role as the biggest frog in its own pond: the human whirlwind named Huey Long had, among other things, given it the competition of an expanded state university in Baton Rouge and a state-supported medical school in New Orleans itself. Hoping for new ideas and (though he claimed otherwise) new sources of money, Jones included on his board of visitors local lawyers and businessmen, an editor of the *Wall Street Journal*, the chairman of the National Science Foundation, and Mississippi's crusading editor and foe of segregation, Hodding Carter.[3]

Before Jones's mind hovered the vision of a Harvard of the South, skimming the cream of the region's best young minds and leaving the average students to be educated by the state institutions. To create a major private university in New Orleans, which lacked great wealth and a strong educational tradition, might seem an unlikely hope. Yet talent had often found a home in a city whose music, food, architecture, and gift for fantasy had long delighted the nation. One of the latest demonstrations that New Orleans could be world-class had come in the field of medicine.[4]

Beginning in 1942, Tulane's Edward William Alton Ochsner had built a Mayo Clinic of the South and christened it with his own name. A medical evangelist, Ochsner attributed his success to "Presbyterian luck." Kindly accident (or predestination) had made him look exactly like the great surgeon he was. His charisma was extraordinary; his charm overwhelming. Aided by gifted associates, he brought top-

2. Phillips interview, 1036. See also Bayne-Jones to Chauncey D. Leake, November 2, 1953, in F-1(L–M), Box 28, SBJC.
3. Jones to Bayne-Jones, November 5, 1953, and *Tulane University: The Board of Visitors, 1955* (N.p., n.d.), both in F-5, Box 28, *ibid.*
4. Address of Welcome: Joseph Merrick Jones, Board of Visitors Meeting, March 25, 26, and 27, 1954, *ibid.* "Harvard of the South" is not a phrase used by Jones, though he states the concept clearly; the phrase was a catchword on campus at the time, used, as a rule, with heavy irony by students and faculty alike.

quality group practice to New Orleans, often in the teeth of hostility from practitioners who saw unfair competition not only in his clinic but in his pursuit of excellence.

A key figure in developing Ochsner's medical empire was Jules Blanc Monroe, a lawyer and a member of the Tulane Board of Administrators. Monroe worshiped Ochsner and shaped university policy to meet the needs of the interlocking organizations—Ochsner Clinic Associates, Ochsner Clinic, Inc., Ochsner Foundation, and Ochsner Foundation Hospital—that Monroe's legal skills had forged to transform a gifted surgeon into an institution.

In consequence, the medical school often seemed to be a subordinate part of the Ochsner empire. Ochsner kept the job, salary, and title of chairman of the department of surgery at Tulane School of Medicine, but the department was little more than an abandoned chrysalis from which the transfigured occupant had flown away. In March, 1955, the board of administrators asked B-J to survey and report upon the school, and to recommend changes. Joseph Merrick Jones also expected him to deal personally with Ochsner, as one medical heavyweight to another. Agreeing, B-J noted that "almost any subject discussed [at Tulane] leads to something about the Ochsner-Tulane affair. . . . I will make this a special part of the survey."[5]

Taking time from his Washington duties, B-J began a series of trips down memory lane. Twice a month he flew to New Orleans to meet his colleagues on the pleasant Uptown campus, with its shrubby oaks, its clutter of buildings in contradictory styles, and its seasonal cicadas. He devoted long hours to the downtown medical school and endured the oppressive, smelly clinics of Charity Hospital. But he also enjoyed luncheons at Commander's Palace, dinners at clubs, chatty evenings with relatives, and nights at the Roosevelt Hotel, where he asked for rooms with a view of the Mississippi River. He invariably flew back to Washington with a full briefcase and much more work to do, all unpaid. Why did he do it?

5. On the Ochsner empire, see John Wilds, *Ochsner's: An Informal History of the South's Largest Private Medical Center* (Baton Rouge, 1985). See also Bayne-Jones's Journal: Survey of Tulane University School of Medicine, 4, in F-8(1), SBJC. For Ochsner's own viewpoint on his dismissal, Bayne-Jones, and Joseph Merrick Jones, see John Wilds and Ira Harkey, *Alton Ochsner, Surgeon of the South* (Baton Rouge, 1990), 191–94.

"You like themes of continuity," he told an interviewer, "and you have one in this case, by blood relationships, intellectual interests, social connections, and all that goes with the place of origin to which a man returns." So B-J labored, and gradually a clear picture emerged of the present state of the school where he had begun the study of medicine forty-five years before.[6]

The basic woe of the prospective Harvard of the South was poverty. In the medical school, both physical plant and professors' pay were in sad shape. The professors had no doubt where money should go first: "*Raising salaries is the primary and fundamental precondition to all future planning at Tulane*," declared the executive faculty. B-J agreed, though as ever he lacked belief in the omnipotence of the so-called bottom line. Board member Darwin Fenner (of Merrill Lynch, Pierce, Fenner & Beane) expected him to "take up the problems of administration and management that he, like all businessmen, thinks are so important." But B-J told Fenner flatly that he did not know "whether a dollar spent for pediatrics is better than a dollar . . . for obstetrics."

Instead he sought a sense of the people who made up the medical school and how they interacted. He found them a varied and interesting lot. Certain types inhabited Tulane: on the one hand, dedicated, contentious people who found refuge in a relatively poor school and took satisfaction in working against the odds; on the other, defeated men who had given up and were simply serving out their time. To the first category belonged the head of the department of neurology and psychiatry—a tall man, full of rangy energy and an arrogance in which B-J detected a hint of defensiveness. Why had he come to Tulane? So that he would have an opportunity to "tell people to go to Hell!" Yet his teaching was superb, and the department had grown "large, vigorous and renowned" under his guidance. Equally able was the head of physiology, Hyman Samuel Mayerson, an old friend and a full-timer competent both in research and teaching. To the company of the defeated

6. Bayne-Jones to Joseph Merrick Jones, April 16, 1955, in F-7(1), Box 28, SBJC; Phillips interview, 1024.

belonged the chairman of microbiology—"a beaten man," in B-J's opinion, whose "Department [is] . . . nearly dead."

At Charity Hospital and neighboring Hutchinson Memorial Clinic, B-J marveled at the variety of clinical material, "probably unmatched elsewhere in the United States," he wrote, for the local combination of poverty and tropical ills formed a rich medical lode. On dismal wooden benches the sick poor waited patiently, black and white; the doctors examined in "miserable hot and dusty" cubicles. Yet in this place so easy to dismiss as a medical refuse heap, B-J found no sense of defeat. The small staff, though overwhelmed by work, was energetic, competent, and cheerful. It was on the comfortable Uptown campus that he met "the magnolia mind," a strain of passivity and vague discontent that reminded him of Chekhov's *Cherry Orchard*.[7]

Overall, he found the School of Medicine unsure of itself and uncertain of its goals. Admissions policy was one issue: Tulane longed for a national student body but still gave preference to young people from New Orleans and the South. Racism was another: segregation was dying, yet the class entering the medical school in September, 1955, numbered 180, of whom 4 were women and none were blacks. The board of visitors urged the University Board of Administrators to end segregation in response to the Supreme Court's 1954 ruling; the medical school faculty agreed but lacked the courage to pass a resolution to the same effect.

Like many other schools B-J had known, Tulane seemingly could not come to grips with its role in teaching and research. Supposedly committed to turning out practitioners, the school for thirty years or more had been evolving into a research institution, depending heavily on the federal government and the foundations. In 1955 the university provided little money for research but paid a toll anyway, because the medical school's deficits were enlarged by the overhead costs of supporting its grants.[8]

Finally, Tulane's relations with local organized medicine were poor. Faculty members told B-J that the Orleans Parish Medical Society

7. Bayne-Jones's Journal, 16–17, 28, 58, 87, 110, 126, 144.
8. *Ibid.*, 24–25, 72; M. E. Lapham, Dean, School of Medicine, to Marion B. Folsom, Secretary, HEW, December 1, 1955, in F-13(3), Box 19, SBJC.

was definitely hostile. Practitioners saw the school as a "great mill" making new specialists who settled in a community already over-stocked; they saw it treating the poor for low fees or none and, like Ochsner, encouraging group practice, the bane of conservatives here as elsewhere. (Feeling on the issue was sometimes virulent; in 1941 each member of the group who formed the original Ochsner Clinic had received from his colleagues in organized medicine a purse containing thirty dimes, payment for a professional Judas.)[9]

Leaving aside for the moment the problem of dealing with organized medicine, B-J and Joseph Merrick Jones agreed that the big issues facing the medical school were its relations with Ochsner and its need for money. Dealing with Ochsner had to be direct and personal, and the job fell to B-J. Of his antagonist's achievements he had no doubt; B-J had nothing but praise for the surgeon's hospital, the care of patients, the research undertakings, and the enthusiastic young investigators who filled the new and shining laboratories. But the contrast with Tulane's department of surgery was painfully evident. "The place seemed dying," wrote B-J, and he agreed with faculty members who told him that "Dr. Ochsner was presiding over the destruction of the Department of Surgery."[10]

The ties between the school and the Ochsner empire remained close and, in B-J's view, not all were strictly ethical. During the days of G.I. benefits after World War II, Ochsner Foundation enrolled promising veterans as fellows and registered them for degrees with the Tulane School of Graduate Education. The fellow paid Tulane tuition, and the school delegated his clinical training to the foundation. "In my opinion," wrote B-J, "there was a bit of a racket in this set-up. Both Tulane and Ochsner were playing a game. Tulane for the money, Ochsner for the derived prestige." Several faculty members regularly

9. Wilds, *Ochsner's: An Informal History*, 30. Such tensions are termed town-gown rivalry by physicians and medical historians; their basis, says a recent writer, "is fundamentally economic. Practicing physicians resent [the fact] that full-time faculty, who derive at least part of their income from the university, compete with them for patients" (Robert G. Petersdorf, "The Town-Gown Syndrome," *Journal of the American Medical Association*, CCLVII [May 8, 1987], 2478).

10. Bayne-Jones to Ochsner, July 28, 1955, in F-7(4), Box 28, SBJC; Bayne-Jones's Journal, 132, 139.

received consultants' fees—which, Tulane salaries being what they were, meant a good deal to them—but seemingly performed no work for their added income. The practice, said B-J, "illustrates well the way in which Ochsner [Foundation] has infiltrated Tulane by a kind of bribery." [11]

By now B-J had pretty clearly formulated his own ideas on the Tulane-Ochsner connection. He first tackled seventy-year-old Jules Blanc Monroe. Though the two had known each other from boyhood, B-J was blunt: if Ochsner did not resign as head of the department of surgery, B-J would recommend publicly that he be asked to do so. Surprisingly, Monroe seemed to accept his conclusion. "He knows very well that he has submitted University policy to the doctors of the Ochsner Foundation," B-J reflected, "and transmitted their decisions to a somewhat over-awed Board of Administrators." B-J softened his tone, and Monroe began to mull over some face-saving plan to spare the doctor and himself embarrassment. Meanwhile, B-J spoke no less candidly to Ochsner himself. [12]

But it was apparently Jones who cleared the way by securing a $750,000 foundation grant for the School of Medicine. At last the school was able to put its department chairmen on full-time, an action that enabled Blanc Monroe and Ochsner to find the face-saving maneuver they had sought. Writing to Joseph Merrick Jones on December 8, Ochsner declared that he had stayed on at Tulane at great personal sacrifice, but that now, with the grant in prospect, he felt at last able to lay his burden down. He tendered his resignation as chairman of the department of surgery, and the Tulane Board accepted. "All was in good taste," said B-J at the time, and years later remembered with satisfaction how "the thing was concluded with bows and an exchange of bouquets, and . . . no thought of pistols and coffee at dawn." [13]

B-J's report on the medical school, issued in March, 1956, recapitulated the views he had formed during his visits to the city. He advised a firm commitment by the school to the more than local role that

11. Bayne-Jones's Journal, 162, 170.
12. *Ibid.*, 223.
13. New York *Times*, November 28, 1955; Bayne-Jones's Journal, 220–21, 229; Phillips interview, 1045.

New Orleans' long involvement with European medicine and its own dependence on northern philanthropy made inevitable. At the same time he suggested a diplomatic approach to the local medical societies, in line with his long-tested ploy of joining the enemy to overcome him. One bit of advice looks amusing in retrospect: B-J favored adding blacks to the student body as soon, he said, as the current excitement over segregation had died down a bit. And he advised a formal, written agreement with the Ochsner Foundation, defining its future relations with Tulane as a first step toward an affiliation that would preserve and enhance the status of both.[14]

No doubt the advice was sound. But the actual future of the school was determined by events in which philanthropy, poverty, and race all played parts. Charity Hospital continued to decay, and during the tenure of Ochsner's successor in the department of surgery it ceased to be "a proper teaching hospital." Fortunately, large gifts by many benefactors enabled the medical school to build its own teaching hospital and to emerge as Tulane Medical Center. The university board of administrators voted $1.5 million to raise faculty salaries; and black students entered at last in 1963, when the university voluntarily desegregated.[15]

In the years that followed, B-J kept his interest in Tulane. He continued to attend the meetings of the board of visitors, drawn as much by his birthplace and his family as by the university. As ever, he enjoyed the clubs, the dining, the southern sense of a present past that is far too intense to be called nostalgia. Gaiety was not absent. B-J remained lively as his eightieth birthday approached, and on one occasion felt obliged to apologize to a woman luncheon guest for behaving "dans une manière que n'étais pas comme il faut pour un veillard ce que je suis"—in a manner that was a bit improper for an old man like himself.

Yet a thread of tragedy had always run through his family's history. Joseph Merrick Jones was the sort of man on whom communities lean, as the city recognized by giving him its ultimate recognition as Rex,

14. Bayne-Jones, *Report of a Survey of the School of Medicine, Tulane University, 1955–1956* (Washington, 1956), 38, 61, 67–68.
15. Oscar Creech, "Retrospect and Prospect," *Bulletin of the Tulane Medical Faculty,* XXII (August, 1963), 217–30; John Duffy, *The Tulane University Medical Center: One Hundred and Fifty Years of Medical Education* (Baton Rouge, 1984), 181, 197–98. See also Meeting of the Executive Faculty of the Tulane University Medical School, June 11, 1956, pp. 4, 8, in F-40, Box 28, SBJC.

King of Carnival. Jones seemed likely to endure for many years, almost a natural formation in the delta landscape. But early on the morning of March 11, 1963, a fire broke out in his comfortable home. His wife was asphyxiated by the smoke, and Jones suffered burns in attempting to rescue her. He died of a heart attack on the way to Ochsner Foundation Hospital, even as Alton Ochsner struggled to save him.

B-J had lost another Joseph Jones, sixty-nine years after the first. This time he well understood that the university and the city grieved with him.[16]

The past returned to B-J in other ways. In retirement he attempted to pursue his long-delayed life of Joseph Jones, but as ever the subject eluded his efforts. Even after so many years, he remained too involved with his grandfather's memory to achieve the distance needed for biography.

Less personal topics were easier to deal with. His friends encouraged him; many of his generation were engaged in literary work, turning out history as a preliminary to becoming history themselves. B-J took a hand during the fifties in establishing the National Library of Medicine on the grounds of the National Institutes of Health in Bethesda. Here he spent much of his later life working on the official histories of the Army Medical Department during World War II. He presided over the series on preventive medicine and contributed a long essay on the Typhus Commission and another on the difficult, complex medical side of civil affairs and military government among newly liberated and newly conquered peoples. But perhaps his most original work was done on a topic that fell to him by chance—the medical treatment of prisoners of war. He soon became aware that American planning and practice in both Europe and North Africa during World War II had been inadequate, in some cases so much so that the field forces could not have lived up to the terms of the Geneva Convention even if they had wished to.[17]

16. Bayne-Jones to Doris H. Austin, May 10, 1963, in F-49, Box 28, SBJC; see also New Orleans *States-Item*, March 11, 1963.

17. See materials in G-24, Box 35, SBJC. Ground for the new library was broken in 1959, and the building was dedicated in 1961, with Bayne-Jones in attendance on both occa-

208

WAR AND HEALING

He talked the problem over with an old friend. Tom Whayne remarked that the "Americans and British did not handle prisoners of war
any worse than anyone else," and advised B-J to write "'just as stark as
it is, and then start from there,'" which sounded like a formula for
ultimate bowdlerization. But B-J was already writing "frankly," as he
said, and the final essay, even if softened in some details (lack of early
drafts makes this impossible to determine) made the basic point with
sometimes devastating candor. (Harking back to Joseph Jones, B-J compared the conditions in one American-run camp in Germany to Andersonville prison in 1864.) His account provided comfort neither for army
publicists nor for the popular notion that the Western Allies had always
been paladins of the humane virtues. But a quarter-century later the
essay remains a convincing account of a little-known subject and an
instructive sidelight on the realities of war.[18]

He also undertook a general introductory essay on the history of
preventive medicine in the army that evolved into a little book. Writing
here of remote as well as contemporary things, he browsed through
rare-book rooms, delighting in the discovery of "new sources, I think,
that haven't been put together," and tasting the scholar's pleasure in
connecting the present to the past. B-J produced a brief but solid work
on his Cinderella specialty and adorned it with pictures of old friends
and heroes—William Crawford Gorgas, William Henry Welch, and
Hans Zinsser.

Published two years before B-J's death, the book, by intention or
not, formed his last tribute to the vision of medicine he had learned and
practiced in war and adopted as a personal faith. The first business of

sions. On the surgeon general's history program, see Albert G. Love, The Historical Division,
August 1, 1941–July 28, 1945, pp. 14–15, in Box 73, SBJC.

18. Minutes of the 9th Meeting, Advisory Editorial Board, June 3, 1957, in Box 57,
SBJC; Bayne-Jones, "Typhus Fever," 176–274. See also Bayne-Jones, Ira V. Hiscock, and
Morrison C. Stayer, "The Americas," Bayne-Jones and Thomas B. Turner, "Planning and
Preparations for the European Theater of Operations," and Bayne-Jones and Edward J.
Dehné, "The European Theater of Operations," all in Civil Affairs/Military Government, ed.
Ebbe Curtis Hoff (Washington, 1976), 59–130, 405–503, Vol. VIII of Hoff, ed., Preventive
Medicine in World War II; and Bayne-Jones, "Enemy Prisoners of War," in Special Fields,
ed. Ebbe Curtis Hoff (Washington, 1968), Vol. IX of Hoff, ed. Preventive Medicine in World
War II.

medicine is health and not disease; the work of keeping people well is as demanding as the work of curing them, and more important. And health means faculties developed and potential fulfilled, "a Greek . . . ideal," rather than a lazy acceptance of the absence of pain.[19]

During his years in Washington, B-J put these and other favored arguments to a variety of audiences, at professional meetings, commencements (he harvested honorary degrees at a great rate), and in many an after-dinner gathering. He gladly played the wise old man; it was honors time in his life, and he accepted whatever scrolls or medals came his way. Most who honored him invited him to speak, and he was happy to do so. He was in demand not only because he was witty and turned a neat compliment to his hosts of the evening but also because his experiences were so wide that he could relate many aspects of medicine to one another. If all else failed, he spoke on Joseph Jones, whose cranky comprehensiveness allowed him to be brought into almost anything.

One continuing theme was the New Humanism. The educated person, B-J believed more deeply than ever, must know something of science and the scientist much of the humanities. He thought more and more of the humanistic medicine of Welch and Osler, with its roots in the long tradition of medical thought as well as in the laboratory. He admired the wholeness of their vision, later broken by the overwhelming accumulation of knowledge and the pride and wealth induced by laboratory triumphs and worldly success.

Speaking to the Medical Writers Institute, he quoted Francis Bacon's lines: "The office of medicine is but to tune this curious harp of man's body and to reduce it to harmony." But to attain a vision of harmony meant seeing man whole, in his context of society and history. In good science writing, "the tuned ear and . . . the eye of imagination" could vividly perceive the background "culture of medicine and war" that embraced and formed the passing event. To the medical writers, dedicated by the nature of their work to the fusion of science with the literary tradition, he gave at the end of his address one of the best of

19. Bayne-Jones, *Evolution of Preventive Medicine*, 1–2; and Major Approaches to Better Health, [March 5, 1957], in I-11, SBJC.

his farewells: "I thank you for listening to me, and I wish you the utmost in craftsmanship."[20]

In 1962 he had a bout of serious illness: streptococci entered his bloodstream during dental work, and the general infection that resulted sent him to Johns Hopkins Hospital, to a pavillion where he had worked as an intern half a century before. Treatment with massive doses of penicillin destroyed the infection, and as he recovered he began to quiz the interns about the history of the hospital. He discovered to his amazement that most had never heard of William Henry Welch. How could the "great founder of the place . . . have passed out of memory," he wondered, and how could the people who held in their hands the future of medicine be made to believe that their calling had a past worth knowing?[21]

Yet he recognized the failings of history, and confessed to a gathering at the Cosmos Club that "there is something inherently dull in the usual academical history of medicine." He disliked the whole process by which the formal superseded the informal; he preferred Osler's method of weaving medical history into his clinical rounds and conveying it with the verve of the great teacher: "wit, puckishness, eloquence and understanding." He hoped for a return to the unity of outlook he associated with the Hippocratic writings, for progress meant not only the uncovering of new truths but the rediscovery of old ones wrongly brushed aside. "The present," he told an audience at Emory University, "is not always modern, and the past may be the really new phenomenon."[22]

The past that he praised and recorded sometimes pressed heavily upon him. One day late in March, 1966, the head of the National Library's

20. Bayne-Jones, The Cultural Background of Medical Writing, September 25, 1964, in I-43, Box 47, SBJC.

21. Phillips interview, 1100.

22. Lecture, Washington Society for the History of Medicine, 1969, and The Consequences of Microbiology for Modern Medicine, address delivered on the occasion of the centennial celebration of the Emory University School of Medicine, Atlanta, October 4, 1954, both in I-5(2), Box 55, SBJC. The second address was later reprinted with emendations in Emory University Quarterly, X (December, 1954), 216–25.

History of Medicine Division entered B-J's study and asked if he would consent to be interviewed by Harlan Phillips. Phillips specialized in oral history and had assembled a book dictated by a man B-J knew well: *Felix Frankfurter Reminisces.* B-J demurred, but not strongly. A few days later he packed his papers—"13 cartons!" he marveled—and workers from the library picked them up. He met Phillips and began talking for the tape recorder on April 11, 1966.[23]

The taping soon turned into a marathon. B-J had lived a long life, and most figures of note in twentieth-century American medicine entered the story at some point. Nan moved through it, honored but guarded by her husband, as did the Baynes, Joneses, and Denegres whose lives had been interwoven with his own. Sometimes he saw his life as happenstance, sometimes as a pattern in which all elements were necessary. The paradox amused him; his philosophy had always been unsystematic. All in all, however, he found his feat of recollection more than he had bargained for, "a severe experience, occupying most of a year. . . . I dictated 7 miles of magnetic tape!"

Though the interviews had not been "Freudian couch affairs," they brought too many things to mind, too many dead friends, too much time gone by, and they left him depressed. Soon he had other reasons for discomfort. In late 1969 he suffered a heart attack; he recovered, but as a markedly slower and older man. He had turned over to others the record of his life that he wished to leave, and he knew that not much time was left.[24]

As soon as he could he returned to his work at the library. On February 20, 1970, he rose as usual, dressed, put on his topcoat, and walked into his living room to wait for a driver the army had allotted him. He sat down in a wing chair at a bay window to keep an eye on the street. When Nan came into the room a few minutes later, she found him dead. She called Walter Reed Army Hospital, then Tom Denegre, and Tom and his wife Louise hurried to her.

---

23. Bayne-Jones to Dr. and Mrs. Iago Galdston, December 30, 1968, Hill to Daniels, January 24, 1968, and Bayne-Jones to Daniels, March 9, 1968, all in I-5(2), Box 55, SBJC.

24. Bayne-Jones to George Denegre II, January 24, 1967, and Bayne-Jones to Joseph Stokes, Jr., July 19, 1967, both in Folder Oral History Memoir (Bayne-Jones—Stokes Material), Box 55, SBJC.

They found Nan sitting in a chair beside B-J's body. For more than two hours, while they waited for the interminably delayed ambulance, Nan chatted like a skilled hostess who feels an obligation to entertain her guests. From time to time she leaned forward and patted B-J's arm. At last the men came from Walter Reed; the body was removed to the hospital, pronounced dead, and an autopsy performed. B-J had died of "acute coronary insufficiency; arteriosclerotic cardiovascular disease."

He was buried at Arlington with military honors. The day was fine despite the month and season, with sunshine and flags snapping in the breeze. From the hillside near President Kennedy's grave the mourners could see the Washington Monument and the Capitol dome through the latticework of wintry branches. Nan endured the ceremony, firm and composed like a military wife.

For weeks afterward, she was kept busy by an avalanche of messages from those who had known B-J, some formal, many personal. Her sister recalled the days when B-J, courting Nan, had taken the two of them sailing on Chesapeake Bay: the sunlight, the smell of the rigging, and how hard he had made them work. Others offered solace according to their own beliefs. The chaplain of Yale spoke the ultimate epitaph for a scientist: "There was nothing true that he was afraid to know."[25]

To sum up neatly a life so long and so complex would be impossible. B-J's career embodied many of the changes that overtook American medicine in the twentieth century. Yet he made each of the roles he played uniquely his own. A medical administrator for much of his professional life, he made no contribution to the theory of management; he specifically rejected most quantitative measures of performance, was inefficient by formal standards, and often failed to meet his budgets. He viewed as mischievous the devices by which bureaucratic managers multiply busywork in the name of improved control. Instead, he tried

25. Interview with Thomas B. and Louise Denegre; Department of the Army, Office of the Adjutant General, Report of Casualty, R-0037, 10 March 1970, in Bayne-Jones's 201 file. See also the Reverend Sidney Lovett to Nan, March 4, 1970, in GDC. Nan died six years later and was buried with her husband.

to get a feel for the people who made an organization work and then sought to liberate them to do whatever they did best. Fundamentally, he knew that his business was not to run organizations but to create the circumstances in which others could teach, research, and heal.

That was his role, the outcome of his personal strengths and weaknesses in the profession that fate and his family had allotted him. By doing what he did best he achieved the success he sought, and something more. He won a solid place among the small group of people who directed the American medical research establishment as it moved toward world leadership. He helped to uphold the institutions he served, and awards from two nations, three armies, and eight universities testified to their gratitude. There were other and deeper benefits. In the process of gaining his hard-earned reputation he liberated himself from the alienage that had darkened his youth. And in performing his proper work he contributed to saving uncounted human lives.

In his own life paradoxes abounded. He devoted endless labor to gaining, and distributing to medical researchers, the largesse of foundations and the government. Yet he viewed the impact of the golden stream with foreboding that sometimes darkened into alarm.. He devoted much of his time on earth to the prevention of disease, and yet he was willing to spread disease, if necessary, through "public health in reverse"—biological warfare. He adopted as a personal credo the view that the finest task of medicine is the active propagation of health, and yet he drew that insight from his own experience of war. Like any administrator, he was a man of his time, responding to the daily crises that form the executive's life. Yet B-J was subject to unworldly longings. He had quaint and durable notions of culture and honor, and an unfashionable faith in the power of life—the subject of the medical art—to subvert all tyrannies, including those of technology and dehumanized science.

To the end of his life he held tenaciously to the things that had formed its beginning. He clung to his family, his roots, and the particular mood and outlook of his generation. Physicians of his time learned a humanistic culture before they learned science, and a theme of B-J's life was his effort to promote that culture of mingled fact and aspiration during a time when it fell into eclipse. He did not despair of its revival, for he had the shrewdness to know that the present may not be modern and that the past may hold the key to the future. He believed firmly that the rediscovery of its past would help to make the medical establishment he served more worthy of its great and ever-growing influence in human affairs.

Selected Bibliography

Manuscripts

Armed Forces Epidemiological Board. Records, 1941–1963. Record Group 334, National Archives and Records Administration, Washington, D.C.

Bayne, Hugh A. Memoirs, 1870–1954. 2 vols. Sterling Memorial Library, Yale University, New Haven.

Bayne-Jones, Stanhope. Army Personnel (201) File, 1914–1971. Federal Personnel Records Center, St. Louis.

———. Collection, 1888–1971. National Library of Medicine, Bethesda, Maryland.

———. Interviews with Harlan B. Phillips, Bethesda, Md., 1967. Transcript in the National Library of Medicine.

Cochrane, Rexmond C. "History of the Chemical Warfare Service in World War II, 1 July 1940–15 August 1945: Biological Warfare Research in the United States." Vol. I of 2 vols. U.S. Army Center of Military History, Washington, D.C.

Fulton, John F. Diary, 1928–1954. Vols. VIII and X. Medical Historical Library, Sterling School of Medicine, Yale University, New Haven.

Jones, Charles C., Jr. Papers, 1865–1893. Louisiana State University Archives, Baton Rouge.

Jones-Denegre-Bayne Collection, 1870–1966. In possession of George Denegre II, New Orleans.

Jones, Joseph. Papers, 1850–1900. Louisiana State University Archives, Baton Rouge.

Presidents of the New York Hospital–Cornell Medical Center. Papers, 1939–1962, and 1945–1975. Medical Archives, New York Hospital–Cornell University Medical Center, New York.

Secretary-Treasurers, New York Hospital–Cornell Medical Center. Papers, 1911–1960, 1927–1978. Medical Archives, New York Hospital–Cornell University Medical Center, New York.

Surgeon General's Office, U.S. Army. Records, 1818–. Record Group 112, National Archives and Record Service, Washington, D.C.

SELECTED BIBLIOGRAPHY

United States of America Typhus Commission. Papers, 1942–1946. National Library of Medicine, Bethesda.
Yale Medical School. Records of the Dean. Yale Archives, Sterling Memorial Library, Yale University, New Haven.

Books

Advancement of Medical Research and Education Through the Department of Health, Education, and Welfare. Washington, 1958.
American Battle Monuments Commission. *26th Division: Summary of Operations in the World War.* Washington, 1944.
Ashburn, P. M. *A History of the Medical Department of the United States Army.* Boston, 1929.
Atwater, Edmund, *et al. To Each His Farthest Star.* Rochester, N.Y., 1975.
Bayne-Jones, Stanhope. *The Evolution of Preventive Medicine in the United States Army, 1607–1939.* Washington, 1968.
———. *Joseph Jones.* N.p., [1957].
———. *Man and Microbes.* Baltimore, 1932.
———. *Report of a Survey of the School of Medicine, Tulane University, 1955–1956.* Washington, 1956.
Becke, Archibald Frank, comp. *Order of Battle of Divisions: Part I, The Regular British Divisions.* London, 1935.
Benison, Saul. *Tom Rivers: Reflections on a Life in Medicine and Science.* Cambridge, Mass., 1967.
Benwell, Harry A. *History of the Yankee Division.* Boston, 1919.
Blackham, Robert J. *Scalpel, Sword and Stretcher: Forty Years of Work and Play.* London, n.d.
Breeden, James O. *Joseph Jones, M.D.: Scientist of the Old South.* Lexington, Ky., [1975].
Butler, Charles Terry. *A Civilian in Uniform.* N.p., 1975.
Cooke, Alistair, ed. *The Vintage Mencken.* New York, 1955.
Chamberlain, Weston P., and Frank W. Weed. *The Medical Department of the United States Army in the World War: Sanitation.* Vol. VI of 15. Washington, 1926.
Chapin, W. A. R. *The Lost Legion.* Springfield, Mass., 1926.

Coffman, Edward M. *The War to End All Wars: The American Military Experience in World War I.* New York, 1968.

Corner, George W. *George Hoyt Whipple and His Friends: The Life-Story of a Nobel Prize Pathologist.* Philadelphia, 1963.

Cowdrey, Albert E. *The Medics' War.* Washington, 1987.

Crile, Grace, ed. *George Crile, An Autobiography.* 2 vols. Philadelphia, 1947.

Crosby, Alfred W. *Epidemic and Peace, 1918.* Westport, Conn., 1976.

Cushing, Harvey. *From a Surgeon's Journal, 1915–1918.* Boston, 1936.

Dowling, Harry F. *Fighting Infection.* Cambridge, Mass., 1977.

Duffy, John. *The Healers: A History of American Medicine.* Urbana, 1976.

Edmonds, James E., ed. *History of the Great War: Military Operations in France and Belgium—1917.* London, 1948.

Flexner, Abraham. *I Remember: The Autobiography of Abraham Flexner.* New York, 1940.

Flexner, Simon, and James Thomas Flexner. *William Henry Welch and the Heroic Age of American Medicine.* 1941, rpr. New York, 1966.

Foster, W. D. *A History of Medical Bacteriology and Immunology.* London, 1970.

Freidson, Eliot. *Profession of Medicine: A Study of the Sociology of Applied Knowledge.* New York, 1975.

Garceau, Oliver. *The Political Life of the American Medical Association.* Hamden, Conn., 1961.

Garrison, Fielding L. *An Introduction to the History of Medicine.* Philadelphia, 1929.

Gorgas, Marie D., and Burton J. Hendrick. *William Crawford Gorgas: His Life and Work.* New York, 1924.

Grissinger, Jay Weir. *Medical Field Service in France.* Washington, 1928.

Harris, Robert, and Jeremy Paxman. *A Higher Form of Killing: The Secret Story of Chemical and Biological Warfare.* New York, 1982.

Hirschfield, Daniel F. *The Lost Reform: The Campaign for Compulsory Health Insurance in the United States from 1932 to 1943.* Cambridge, Mass., 1970.

Hoff, Ebbe Curtis, ed. *Civil Affairs/Military Government.* Washington, 1976. Vol. VIII of Hoff, ed., *Preventive Medicine in World War II.* 9 vols.

Jackson, Joy. *New Orleans in the Gilded Age: Politics and Urban Progress, 1880–1896.* Baton Rouge, 1969.

SELECTED BIBLIOGRAPHY

Jones, Joseph. *Medical and Surgical Memoirs*. . . . 4 vols. New Orleans, 1876–1890.

Kelley, Brooks Mather. *Yale: A History*. New Haven, 1974.

Larrabee, Eric. *The Benevolent and Necessary Institution: The New York Hospital, 1771–1971*. New York, 1971.

Lechevalier, Hubert A., and Morris Solotorovsky. *Three Centuries of Microbiology*. New York, 1965.

Ludmerer, Kenneth M. *Learning to Heal: The Development of American Medical Education*. New York, 1985.

Melosh, Barbara. *"The Physician's Hand" : Work Culture and Conflict in American Nursing*. Philadelphia, 1982.

Millett, Allan R., and Peter Maslowski. *For the Common Defense: A Military History of the United States of America*. New York, 1984.

Myers, Robert Manson, ed. *The Children of Pride*. Abr. ed. New Haven, 1984.

Numbers, Ronald L. *Almost Persuaded: American Physicians and Compulsory Health Insurance, 1912–1920*. Baltimore, 1978.

Oren, Dan A. *Joining the Club: A History of Jews at Yale*. New Haven, 1985.

Patterson, James T. *The Dread Disease: Cancer and Modern American Culture*. Cambridge, Mass., 1987.

Raynack, Elton. *Professional Power and American Medicine: The Economics of the American Medical Association*. Cleveland, 1967.

Reverby, Susan M. *Ordered to Care: The Dilemma of American Nursing, 1850–1945*. Cambridge, Mass., 1987.

Shryock, Richard H. *American Medical Research Past and Present*. 1947; rpr., New York, 1980.

Siler, Joseph F. *The Medical Department of the United States Army in the World War: Communicable Diseases*. Vol. IX of 15 vols. Washington, 1928.

Smoking and Health: Report of the Advisory Committee to the Surgeon General of the Public Health Service. Washington, [1964].

Starr, Paul. *The Social Transformation of American Medicine*. New York, 1982.

Stewart, Irving. *Organizing Scientific Research for War: The Administrative History of the Office of Scientific Research and Development*. Boston, 1948.

Strode, George K., ed. *Yellow Fever.* New York, 1951.

Thomas, Lewis. *The Youngest Science: Notes of a Medicine-Watcher.* New York, 1983.

U.S. Army Activities in the United States Biological Warfare Programs, 1942–1977. 2 vols. Washington, 1977.

Valenstein, Elliot S. *Great and Desperate Cures: The Rise and Decline of Psychosurgery and Other Radical Treatments for Mental Illness.* New York, 1986.

White, Andrew Dickson. *A History of the Warfare of Science with Theology.* New York, 1896.

Wilds, John. *Ochsner's: An Informal History of the South's Largest Private Medical Center.* Baton Rouge, 1985.

Wilds, John, and Ira Harkey. *Alton Ochsner, Surgeon of the South.* Baton Rouge, 1990.

Zinsser, Hans. *As I Remember Him: The Biography of R. S.* Boston, 1940.

———. *Rats, Lice and History.* Boston, 1935.

Articles

Bayne-Jones, Stanhope. "Board for the Investigation and Control of Influenza and Other Epidemic Diseases in the Army." *Army Medical Bulletin,* No. 64 (October, 1942), 1–22.

———. "The Consequences of Microbiology for Modern Medicine." *Emory University Quarterly,* X (1954), 219–25.

———. "Enemy Prisoners of War." In *Special Fields,* edited by Ebbe Curtis Hoff. Washington, 1968. Vol. IX of Hoff, ed., *Preventive Medicine in World War II.* 9 vols.

———. "Freedom Inherent in Medicine and Physicians." *Diplomate,* XXII (1951), 93–96.

———. "The Hospital as a Center of Preventive Medicine." *Annals of Preventive Medicine,* XXXI (1949), 7–16.

———. "The Outbreak of Jaundice in the Army." *Journal of the American Medical Association,* CXX (1942), 51–53.

———. "Reciprocal Effects of the Relationship of Bacteriology and Medicine." *Journal of Bacteriology,* XXI (1931), 61–73.

SELECTED BIBLIOGRAPHY

————. "A Teacher by Preference." *Science*, CXLIII (1964), 347.

————. "Typhus Fever." In *Communicable Diseases*, edited by Ebbe Curtis Hoff. Washington, 1964. Vol. VII of Hoff, ed., *Preventive Medicine in World War II*. 9 vols.

————. "The United States of America Typhus Commission." *Army Medical Bulletin*, No. 68 (July, 1943), 8.

————. "The Yale University School of Medicine: The Educational Program for a Technical and Idealistic Profession." *Yale Scientific Magazine* (Fall, 1936), n.p.

"Cancer: The Great Darkness." *Fortune*, XV (March, 1937), 112–13, 162–79.

Cowdrey, Albert E. "'Germ Warfare' and Public Health in the Korean Conflict." *Journal of the History of Medicine and Allied Sciences*, XXXIX (April, 1984), 153–72.

Deignan, Stella Leche, and Esther Miller. "The Support of Research in Medical and Allied Fields for the Period 1946 Through 1951." *Science*, CXV (1952), 336.

Foster, Gaines M. "Typhus Disaster in the Wake of War: The American Polish Relief Expedition, 1919–1920." *Bulletin of the History of Medicine*, LV (1981), 221–32.

Fox, Daniel M. "The Politics of the NIH Extramural Program, 1937–1950." *Journal of the History of Medicine and Allied Sciences*, XLII (1987), 447–66.

Fox, John P. "Immunization Against Epidemic Typhus." *American Journal of Tropical Diseases and Hygiene*, V (1956), 464–79.

Grenoilleau, G. "L'Epidemie de typhus en Algerie (1941–1942–1943)." *Archives de l'Institut Pasteur d'Algerie*, XXII (1944), 353–79.

Magasanik, Boris. "Research on Bacteria in the Mainstream of Biology." *Science*, CCXL (1988), 1435–39.

Miller, Lois Mattox, and James Monohan. "The Cigarette Controversy: A Storm Is Brewing." *Reader's Digest*, August, 1963, pp. 91–99.

Petersdorf, Robert G. "The Town-Gown Syndrome." *Journal of the American Medical Association*, CCLVII (1987), 2478–79.

Pressman, Jack D. "John F. Fulton and the Origins of Psychosurgery." *Bulletin of the History of Medicine and Allied Sciences*, LXII (1988), 1–22.

Robbins, Jhan, and June Robbins. "The Great Untold Story of Senator

Robert Taft: Eight Weeks to Live." *New York Herald-Tribune*, January 17, 1954, *The Week* (magazine), pp. 8–9.

Scheele, Leonard A. "A General View of Cancer Research: The Fourth James Ewing Memorial Lecture." *Bulletin of the New York Academy of Medicine*, 2nd ser., XXV (1949), 671–97.

Shannon, James A. "The National Institutes of Health: Some Critical Years, 1955–1957." *Science*, CCXXXVIII (1987), 865–68.

Strong, Richard P. "Hans Zinsser: Bacteriologist, Teacher, Philosopher, Author, Poet, Soldier." *Science*, XCII (1940), 276–79.

Viseltear, Arthur. "Milton C. Winternitz and the Yale University Institute of Human Relations: A Brief Chapter in the History of Social Medicine." *Yale Journal of Biology and Medicine*, LVII (1984), 869–889.

Whipple, George H. "Autobiographical Sketch." *Perspectives in Biology and Medicine*, II (1959), 253–87.

Winternitz, Milton C. "The Institute of Human Relations at Yale University." *New England Journal of Medicine*, CCII (1930), 57.

———. "A New Educational Pattern." *Clinical Medicine and Surgery*, XXXVIII (1931), 473–75.

———. "A Physician Looks at Mental Hygiene." *Mental Hygiene*, XVI (1932), 221–32.

Woodward, T. E., and W. D. Tigertt. "Review of the Activities of the Commission on Epidemiological Survey." *Military Medicine*, CXXVI (1961), 37–39.

Wyngaarden, James B. "The National Institutes of Health in Its Centennial Year." *Science*, CCXXXVIII (1987), 869–74.

Newspapers

Boston *Globe*, March 21, 1936.
Chicago *Daily News*, January 30, 1942.
London *Times*, May 24, 1917.
New Haven *Evening Register*, June 21, 1939.
New Orleans *Daily States*, March 29, 1883.
New Orleans *States-Item*, March 11, 1963.
New York *Herald Tribune*, November 21, 1948.
New York *Times*, 1917–1967.

SELECTED BIBLIOGRAPHY

The Ojai (Nordhoff, Calif.), February 9, 1907.
Paris *Journal de Debats*, June 30, 1932.
Washington *Evening Star*, July 27, 1953, July 1, 1956.
Washington *Post*, March 15, 1970.
New Haven *Yale News*, February 16, 1940.

Index